Bright Line Eating

The Complete Bright Line Eating Cookbook | Delicious, Simple, and Quick Bright Line Eating Recipes For Smart People

Table of Contents

Introduction

The Bright Line Eating method of weight loss is an innovative new approach to nutrition that aims to give participants unprecedented control over their eating habits. The method, which was developed by psychologist Susan Peirce Thompson, uses a model similar to those used to treat substance addiction. Because it uses a simple collection of no-nonsense guidelines to control a participant's eating behavior, the method can be easier to understand and adopt than many more complicated diet plans. And because an easy plan is often easier to stick with, Bright Line Eating claims to be better at truly changing the behavior of its adherents over the long term than other, more convoluted approaches.

In this book, we'll give you a thorough overview of the Bright Line Eating method, its history, the science behind it, its advantages over other diet plans, its approach to nutrition and exercise, and its odds of success.

Most importantly, we'll give a collection of recipes that will help you, if you so choose, to make Bright Line Eating the easy-to-follow basis of your daily meal plans.

Bright Line Eating: An Overview

The Bright Line Eating method is a plan for controlling unhealthy eating habits and losing weight that was developed by psychologist and neuroscientist Dr. Susan Peirce Thompson. The method is outlined and explained in Thompson's bestselling 2017 book, *Bright Line Eating: The Science of Living Happy, Thin, and Free*, and it is supported by a collection of online products aimed at supporting followers.

The Bright Line method is based on both Thompson's personal experience and with her research in the fields of neurobiology and psychology. The method takes as it model the idea that unhealthy eating habits are often the result of food addiction and that the best to modify those unhealthy behaviors is to treat them in the same way that other substance-abuse addictions are often treated.

The core principle behind Bright Line Eating, and the concept from which it gets its name, is the assertion that most diet and weight-loss plans fail because they depend on the dieter to make choices and decisions within the framework of the diet. Furthermore, these diets need the dieter to exercise willpower in order to overcome the urges that lead to unhealthy eating.

Thompson argues that food addicts are not capable of exercising the willpower required to steer clear of unhealthy eating, and that asking them to try is to set them up for failure. Instead, the Bright Line Eating method tries to remove the need for decisions and choices in the meal-planning process by setting up a handful of rules, known as "bright line rules," that are unambiguous, strict, and unbreakable. By establishing a series of bright lines that the dieter cannot, under any circumstances, cross, the responsibility for making food decisions is taken out of the hands of the dieter, and the chances of success for the diet are increased.

Who Is Susan Peirce Thompson?

Susan Peirce Thompson Ana Fleischman in 1974 in Petaluma, California, the daughter of Joseph Carl Fleischman and Mary Peirce. Thompson would eventually drop her father's surname and take both her mother's maiden name and her husband's surname as her own.

As Thompson explains in Bright Line Eating, she was an adventurous kid who lived her early life with lots of energy but not much structure. She describes her childhood as unremarkable until, at the age of 12, she started to combat what she saw as problematic weight gain by dieting.

Thompson's early experiments with dieting were unsuccessful, and she says that at age 14, she began to experiment with drugs, which led to weight loss, but also to addiction. She battled addiction to multiple drugs throughout her teen years, and she dropped out of high school.

In 1994, at the age of 19, Thompson entered her first 12-step program, and she credits that program with her being able to successfully fend off addiction to drugs. With that addiction under control, she was able to return to school, and she received an undergraduate degree in cognitive science from the University of California Berkeley. From there, she went on to a PhD program at the University of Rochester in New York. She also married David Thompson in 1999.

Despite these successes, however, Thompson says that she was still struggling. She battled depression, and she was also once again having trouble controlling her weight. She tried antidepressants and therapy, but nothing was working.

In 2003, Thompson entered another 12-step program, this one focused on helping addicts overcome addiction to food. She lost 60 pounds within months, and her depression went away.

In the meantime, Thompson finished her PhD program, and she went on to a fellowship at an Australian university and two Assistant Professorships at colleges in the United States. By 2016, she had gained tenure in one of those positions but had moved on to an adjunct position back at the University of Rochester.

Through all of her rollercoaster experiences with addiction, weight gains and depression, Thompson became convinced that her knowledge of neurobiology and 12-step programs could be pulled together to create a weight-loss program that would work for those who had struggled on every other kind of diet. In 2014, she developed the Bright Line Eating method.

Food Addiction and Its Consequences

The foundation of Bright Line Eating relies on the concept of food addiction. Far from simple overeating or bad food habits, food addiction is characterized by compulsive eating of food--especially those kinds of food that are high and sugar and fat and are therefore the most psychologically rewarding to eat--to excess, despite the obvious negative consequences that come about from overeating.

Food addicts often engage in binge eating, meaning that they eat large amounts of food in short amounts of time, and they typically feel like they are powerless to stop eating. Even worse, after food binges, food addicts often feel profound feelings of guilt and depression. Very often, these negative feelings lead, eventually, to more bingeing. During extreme binges, a food addict may consume between 5,000 and 15,000 calories, or several times the total daily suggested calorie intake for an adult.

Food addicts also commonly engage in "grazing" behavior, in which they eat at a slower rate between meals, sometimes nearly constantly throughout the day. The calorie content of the foods taken in through individual grazing events is usually a lot less than the calories consumed during a binge, but the cumulative calorie intake can actually be quite large.

The net result for food addicts is that they consume many times more calories than they should, and they often have no clear idea of how much they're eating during the day. Nor do they feel that they have any personal ability to change the way they're eating.

The Bright Line Susceptibility Scale

Thompson's research--as well as her own experience and her intuition--told her that food addiction was the cause of weight gain for many people. She was also certain that her knowledge of neurobiology could help her find a way to confront food addiction that would free food addicts from the compulsions that made them overeat.

Thompson, first of all, developed a quiz that would help determine whether a given dieter was likely to be a food addict and whether, consequently, the Bright Line Eating method had a good chance of being successful for them. The results of the quiz show where the quiz-taker falls on a Susceptibility Scale, a measure of how susceptible the eater is to engaging in food-addict behavior.

The quiz asks questions about the eater's ability to control eating during times of psychological stress, how often the eater feels satisfied after eating, how often the eater craves certain foods, how often the eater thinks about food, and whether the eater has engaged in binge eating during times of stress.

The results of the quiz place the potential dieter on a spectrum, at one end of which is the extreme danger of addict behavior. Dieters on this end of the spectrum are most likely to benefit from a plan like the Bright Line Eating method, Thompson claims. Dieters on the other end of the spectrum are unlikely to be food addicts and may be able to benefit from other weight-loss plans. Thompson says, however, that as many as a third of Americans would score on the high end of the Susceptibility Scale and therefore potentially benefit from a plan like Bright Line Eating.

Drawing the Bright Lines

Bright Line Eating draws its bright lines to specifically address the core problematic behaviors of food addicts. In particular, the method confronts the problems of binge eating, grazing, and the lack of awareness of food consumption. It does so by laying out unambiguous rules that plan adherents are required to follow, without exception or question. The goal is to remove choices and judgment calls from the process of eating, so that food addicts are not asked to rely on their own willpower or decision-making ability.

The Bright Line Eating method establishes four bright lines that may not be crossed under any circumstances. They are:

- No sugar
- No flour
- Three meals a day, and no eating between meals
- Carefully controlled food quantities during meals

The method comes at the problem of binge eating from a couple of different directions. First of all, it specifically prohibits the types of foods that are most likely to be consumed during binges. The prohibition on sugar rules out candies, sweets, cookies, sugary drinks and other high-calorie treats, and the prohibition on flour also outlaws bread, pastries, cakes, pasta and crackers. All of these foods are not only calorie dense, they're also the kinds of food that trigger neurobiological responses in eaters' brains that encourage overindulgence.

The careful control of food quantities also takes on the problem of bingeing. Eaters must weigh all of their food during meals, and they must, without exception, adhere to the limits specified for each type of food. There is no estimation of quantities, and there is no flexibility in the amount of food that can be eaten.

The requirement that BLE adherents eat scheduled meals and may not eat anything at any other time is aimed at controlling grazing. There is no gray area defining when you can eat. You must eat at meal times--no skipping meals--and you may not eat at any other time. Period. Grazing is impossible, and you don't have to wonder if it's all right to eat something--even just a little bit--right now. If it's not meal time, the answer is no.

And, of course, all of the rules help the BLE eater to be keenly aware of what and how much he or she is eating. Everything is precisely controlled, and there's no way for unintended calories to slip under the radar.

Finally, Thompson pulls neurobiology into the equation by suggesting that food addicts have built a resistance to a hormone called leptin, which triggers a feeling of being satisfied after eating when it's released into the bloodstream. Because addicts don't feel the effects of leptin, they tend to feel perpetually hungry, and they have little incentive to stop eating. Thompson claims that adherence to the program's rules causes the brain to "rewire" and once again be receptive to the effects of leptin.

The rationale for this rigorousness in the program grows out of Thompson's experience with 12-step addiction programs. The approach of those programs depends on the application of unambiguous, zero-tolerance rules. An addiction program would never tell an alcoholic that it was fine to have a little drink now and then or tell a heroin addict that using the drug occasionally was okay. These programs do not count on addicts to be able to control their addictions, and Thompson doesn't believe that food addicts should be asked to have that kind of responsibility, either.

How Bright Line Works

Bright Line Eating functions like a 12-step program in other ways, too, in that it relies on building a support system that helps adherents stick to the program's rules. It does so through a series of online products which deliver support, information and materials to subscribers with the goal of introducing initial weight loss, changing eating habits, and offering ongoing support to sustain the new habits.

The first, and most substantial, of the products is the Bright Line Eating Boot Camp. This program lasts for eight weeks and includes support in the form of a dedicated meal plan, educational video modules, online support groups, weekly coaching calls, and other support materials.

Thompson claims that the average weight loss for Boot Camp participants is 17 pounds and that weight losses in excess of 25 pounds in eight weeks is not uncommon.

Bright Line Eating also offers a condensed version of the Boot Camp, called the 14-Day Challenge, which offers some of the same support in a limited way. This program is geared toward participants who are unsure whether or not the program will work for them or who are not ready to make the substantial financial investment required by the Boot Camp.

An ongoing support program, called Bright Lifers, that's intended to support BLE participants after they've completed the Boot Camp. This program includes an online support community, daily Accountability Calls, access to the program's educational archives, and discounts on other products.

Bright Line Food Requirements

The food requirements for Bright Line Eating are both extremely simple and extremely restrictive. There are only two categories of foods that are strictly prohibited, but those two categories of ingredients are present in a bewildering array of foods.

First of all, Bright Line Eating prohibits sugar. That may sound like a simple prohibition, but it extends beyond the processed granulated white sugar that probably comes immediately to mind when you hear the word. You can't eat that kind of sugar, but you also can't eat natural, unprocessed or minimally processed sugars such as honey, agave, or maple syrup.

You also can't eat fruit products that concentrate natural fruit sugars. That includes fruit juices and dried fruits, although whole, fresh fruit is allowed.

Don't think you'll be able to replace sugar with artificial sweeteners, either. Sweeteners such as stevia, sucralose, aspartame, saccharin and the like are prohibited, too.

The story with flour is much the same. Processed white wheat flour is prohibited, as is whole wheat flour. But also prohibited are any other flours, such as oat flour, buckwheat flour, rice flour, almond flour, or coconut flour.

Bright Line Eating doesn't prohibit all these foods just to be mean. It has, instead, to do with neurobiology. When we consume sugars and processed flours, we get a strong positive reaction psychologically thanks to the release of a hormone called dopamine, so over time, food addicts can become conditioned to crave that dopamine jolt. By cutting out the foods that cause a spike in dopamine, the BLE plan tries to get dopamine cravings under control.

Bright Line and Nutrition

Often when diets restrict access to certain categories of foods, they do so at the expense of complete nutrition. Low-carb diets, for example, severely limit the consumption of carbohydrates, a key macronutrient that is vital to healthy bodily function. If the restriction is taken too far, it can have an adverse effect on a dieter's overall health.

Bright Line Eating, however, doesn't necessarily endanger a dieter's adherence to proper, complete nutrition. Its restrictions on sugar and flour place limits on carbohydrate consumption, but participants still have plenty of access to other sources of carbohydrates, and those source of unprocessed carbs are likely healthier sources, anyway.

In addition, the removal of so many processed carbs from the participant's diet encourage their replacement with other foods that are higher in other nutrients, such as fiber, protein, and even fat.

Bright Line vs Other Diets

As we've said before, the principal difference between Bright Line Eating and most other diet plans is that BLE does not ask its participants to make any choices. Most other plans, even strict low-carb diets, build some flexibility into their plans. In most plans, you can eat virtually anything in moderation, and it's up to you to put limits on yourself to keep yourself on the plan.

Bright Line Eating acknowledges that some people simply aren't capable of dealing with that kind of freedom. They need a plan that tells them, unequivocally, when they can eat, what they can eat, and how much they can eat.

Thompson admits that not everyone needs quite so much regimentation in their diet plan, and those people who do not score high on the Susceptibility Scale may be able to successfully lose weight on a more flexible plan and, more importantly, keep it off.

Bright Line Eating and Exercise

Thompson and the Bright Line Eating plan have a somewhat controversial stance when it comes to dieting and exercise. While most diet and nutrition plans stress the importance of being physically active while trying to lose weight, Thompson argues that exercising during a weight-loss plan is actually counterproductive.

Thompson claims, among other things, that exercise makes room for excuses during a weight-loss plan. If you exercise, you're likely to think that you're entitled to eat more in compensation for the physical activity.

Thompson also argues that the mental and psychological effort required to begin an exercise plan takes important focus away from the job of changing your eating habits. Willpower is a finite resource, she says, and if you use up your willpower on making yourself go to the gym, you're more likely to fail when you need willpower to eat better.

Because of these arguments, Thompson says that dieters should only think about starting to exercise after they've already lost weight and have successfully changed their eating habits.

Is There a Downside to BLE?

The most common criticism of the Bright Line Eating program, by far, is its cost. The BLE Boot Camp initially had a very steep price of almost $1,000 for the eight-week program. That cost has since been reduced by about half, which still makes it nearly $500. The 14-Day Challenge is available for $29, but that program is intended as an introduction and is designed to lead into the Boot Camp. Ongoing support doesn't come cheap, either, with membership in Bright Lifers and the purchase of other products potentially costing hundreds of dollars per year.

Although Bright Line Eating is generous with the amount of information and educational resources it makes available for free, fully detailed eating plans, access to extensive archives, and online support is available only to paying members.

The high cost of the program has led some to be critical of Thompson's incorporation of the principles of other food-addiction recovery programs whose resources are free. Thompson admits that the BLE method is based heavily on a 12-step program such as Foods Addicts in Recovery Anonymous, and she recommends that program for food addicts who can't afford the BLE products.

A Few Things to Remember

This collection of recipes is meant to support followers of the Bright Line Eating plans, but it is not an official product of Bright Line Eating. These recipes are designed to fit within the guidelines and restrictions of the plan, but they were not created, designed or endorsed by the Bright Line organization itself. Although we've made every effort to include recipes that fit well within the confines of the Bright Line Eating philosophy, we can't guarantee that they will always conform to the rules or requirements of every Bright Line Eating plan.

That being said, we encourage you to use the recipes to help you make your Bright Line

Eating plan a success, but you should always be aware of the specific requirements and needs of your own personalized plan. Everyone's needs are different, and you'll likely need to make adjustments to the recipes in order to fit them within your own plan boundaries. We've designed the recipes and their presentation to make that kind of adjustment as easy as possible, but it's ultimately up to you to make sure that you're staying true to your plan. Know what the requirements and prohibitions of your specific plan are, and ensure that every recipe is consistent with them before you include that recipe in your meal planning.

Don't forget, too, that the quantities, cooking and preparation times, and ingredient choices are estimates, and you might need to make adjustments to them, too, to get the most from the recipes. If you do substitute ingredients or adjust quantities, though, be sure to note the changes and be aware of whether or not the adjustments adhere to your plan.

Finally, we want to caution you to take your general physical health into account before you embark on a Bright Line Eating plan, or any diet plan, for that matter. The Bright Line Eating plan in particular is very restrictive in what it does and does not allow you to eat, and before you take the leap and change your eating habits to conform to the plan, you need to know whether or not it will have an adverse effect on your health.

Also, Bright Line's controversial views on physical activity make it a poor fit for some people with particular health concerns. A Bright Line Eating plan is sometimes seen as a license for physical inactivity, and that might not be a good choice for you to make, especially if you have health issues that are exacerbated by low levels of activity and exercise.

Before you make radical changes to the way you eat, or to your physical activity level, you should consult with a physician, nutritionist, or other health care professional to find out if the changes are safe for you to pursue.

Recipes

Probably the most challenging part of staying on a Bright Line Eating plan is finding interesting foods to eat that stay within the boundaries of the plan but that still keep you satisfied. One of the best ways to keep yourself happy with your diet plan is to ensure that you stay positive about eating and that you appreciate the food you eat for what it is, rather than something you wish it was. With that in mind, we've collected recipes that are far from ordinary, that use flavors and ingredients in new ways, and that are likely to keep you upbeat and excited during meal times. Our goal is to give you food options that will make you feel like your Bright Line Eating plan is an adventure, not an ordeal.

You'll notice that many of our recipes are built around plant-based ingredients, and they find protein sources other than meat. There are a couple of reasons for that. First of all, we understand the challenges of creating a varied, interesting menu within the Bright Line framework. Meats are easy; since they aren't restricted by any of the Bright Line rules, basic meat dishes are unlikely to run afoul of your plan.

Plant-based dishes are often trickier. The prohibition of flour, of course, rules out pastas, breads, and other flour-based staples that form the foundation of many non-meat dishes. As you're trying to build a meal plan, you'll probably often run into the problem of a dish that would be perfect except for one problematic ingredient that's indispensable to the recipe.

We've tried to find a way around that problem by giving you a collection of plant-based recipes that will augment your favorite meats and meat dishes, and you won't have to sacrifice any flavor by substituting or subtracting ingredients that are not Bright Line-friendly.

Secondly, we know that there's a temptation to avoid the problem altogether by relying too much on meat-based dishes. That's not a great idea, because it undermines the goal of balanced nutrition in your diet, and it also sets you up to eventually get bored and unhappy with your meal planning. Our recipe collection is designed to keep your daily menu planning full of spice, variety, and complete, balanced nutrition. You'll get plenty of crucial nutrients from plant-based sources, and you'll get some of the essential nutrients you lose by eliminating flour by eating plenty of allowable grains. You might even find that the alternative sources of protein offered in our collection will lead you to reducing that amount of meat in your weekly diet.

That's not to say that we're trying to get you to eliminate meat from your diet. We've included meat dishes that fit well within the Bright Line framework, and we encourage you to use them to keep your meal planning interesting.

Understanding the Recipes

We've structured our recipes in a consistent, informative way that will help you incorporate them into your own personal Bright Line Eating plan. Everyone who approaches Bright Line is going to do so a little bit differently, so we've tried to give you the information you need in each recipe to be able to adapt the dishes to fit your own personalized requirements.

With that in mind, here's a guide to all the information that's included with each recipe, so you can get the most from each one and make the dishes perfectly suited to the unique needs of your plan.

Servings and Time Required

Some of the recipes are designed so that they make an individual serving that's perfectly right for you to make and eat in a single meal. That's an advantage over typical recipes, which might require you to do tricky math or division of ingredients to figure out what a single serving consists of.

Other recipes don't work as well in single-serving sizes, so we've included the total number of servings produced by each recipe. We've tried, though, in these cases to make it easy to understand what makes up an individual serving so that you can more easily know how much of the recipe you can eat in a single meal. The rest of the recipe can be shared with friends or family, or, in many cases, the leftovers can be saved for another meal.

The time required to make each recipe is important, obviously, because we know that you're busy and you probably don't want to spend too much of your time with meal preparation. Many of the recipes in the collection are quick and easy to put together, and if they take a little longer to prepare, we're going to warn you right up front. Keep in mind that our time requirements are only estimates; you might be able to finish them faster if you're a speedy cook!

Components of Each Serving

Here's where we get down to the nitty gritty of what makes up each recipe. As you work on your Bright Line Eating plan, you're going to need to keep track of the components of your meal planning, and you're going to need to measure and track your consumption of vegetables, fruits, proteins, grains, and fats. In conventional recipes, all of these components are hidden in the ingredient lists, and it's not easy to sort out where each of the categories is lurking in the dish and how much of each is in there.

To help you solve that problem, we've broken out each component of each dish so you know what makes up the totality of the recipe. We'll tell you before you even get started how many servings of fruit, vegetables, protein, fat and grains are in each individual serving, even if the entire recipe makes more than one serving. That way, after you've divided the final product, you know how much of each component you're getting in an individual serving.

Don't forget, however, that we're using standard serving-size measurements that might not necessarily correspond with the requirements of your personal plan. In general, we've stuck with four-ounce servings sizes for most of the components, and we'll usually instruct you to weigh and measure ingredients to conform to your plan at the stage when measurement is important.

Ingredients for Each Component

This is another way in which our recipes differ greatly from the structure of typical cookbook recipes. Traditionally, ingredient lists lay out the ingredients you need in the order you need them in the recipe. That makes sense from the perspective of workflow in the kitchen; you can see what you need when you need it.

When it comes to Bright Line Eating, however, that kind of organization can be a little confusing. You might throw in a vegetable ingredient here, a fat or protein there, and then a grain or fruit. Before you know it, everything is mixed up together, and you have no idea what is actually in your dish and how much of it is there.

That's why we've broken the ingredient lists out by component, so that you can understand where you're vegetables, fruits, grains, proteins and fats are coming from. We've grouped the ingredients together by category so that you can track them more easily, and you can much more easily make adjustments as you need to in order to fit each recipe into your personalized plan.

Other Ingredients

What about those pesky ingredients that don't fit into any of the main Bright Line categories? These ingredients are grouped together at the end of ingredients list. These ingredients include spices, condiments, and other items that don't count against your main plan component limits; they are, essentially, freebies. We've also included here optional ingredients that you can chose to leave out or to adjust quantities as you're able to do so within your plan.

Additions for Those on Maintenance Plans

We want the recipes to be as flexible as possible so that you can use them no matter what stage of your Bright Line Eating journey you're currently in. The recipes are designed from the start to be usable by those who are using Bright Line Eating to get their eating habits under control and to lose weight, so we've structured them as rigidly as possible.

More advanced Bright Line eaters who are no longer trying to lose weight and are on longer-term maintenance plans are likely to be able to eat more and more varied versions of the same recipes. To assist these eaters, we've included in many of the recipes suggestions for how you can bump up the ingredient lists, serving sizes or accompaniment for the dishes to take advantage of the modified requirements for maintenance plans.

Directions

Now that you understand all the supporting information for each recipe, it's time to get into the kitchen and get started. We've made the directions for each dish as clear and concise as possible, and we've chosen recipes that even novice cooks can understand and pull off with ease.

Breakfast

We all know that breakfast is the most important meal of the day, and you should never skip it, no matter what sort of diet plan you're following. When you're on a Bright Line Eating plan, however, there is no choice; the requirement for three meals a day is a non-negotiable bright line, and you must eat a real meal to begin your day.

Of course, it's never easy to put together a well-balanced meal first thing in the morning, especially one that adheres to the strict Bright Line guidelines. To help you out, we've included here a few recipes that will get you going on your way with a solid serving of grains and fruits or vegetables, and they don't require huge amounts of preparation. One of the recipes is a Bright-Line-compliant version of one of the oldest breakfast staples on any menu, oatmeal. Another is a variation on a grain-based breakfast that rests on a non-traditional foundation of quinoa.

And, finally, we're including a quiche-like treat that serves up a delightfully filling breakfast without depending on a forbidden pastry crust. This one takes a little longer to prepare, but if you plan ahead and make it the night before, it makes a delicious breakfast the next morning (or even the morning after that).

Cinnamon-Apple Cereal

Number of Servings: Makes 1 Serving

Time Required: About 30 minutes

Components of Each Serving:

- Grain Servings: 1
- Protein Servings: 1
- Fruit Servings: 1

Ingredients:

Fruit Component:

- 1 diced apple

Protein Component:

- 1 oz. nuts or nut butter
- 4 oz. of low fat or skim milk or yogurt

Grain Component:

- 1 oz. dry quinoa (makes 4 oz. of cooked quinoa)

Other ingredients:

- 4 oz. water (½ cup)
- ½ tsp. cinnamon
- A pinch each of nutmeg, allspice, cloves, cardamom

Additions for Those on Maintenance Plans:

- *Grain Component:* Increase quinoa to 1 ½ oz. and water to ¾ cup.
- *Protein Component:* Increase nuts/nut butter to 2 oz. and milk/yogurt to 8 oz.

Directions:

1. Measure out 1 ounce of quinoa into a small sauce pan with a lid.

2. Add the diced apple, water, and spices.

3. Cover the pan and bring it to a simmer over medium-low heat. Simmer for about 20 minutes, or until all the water is absorbed.

4. The quinoa cereal can be stored in the refrigerator, in a tightly sealed container, for a 3-5 days.

Bright Oatmeal

Number of Servings: Makes 1 Serving

Time Required: About 20 minutes

Components of Each Serving:

- Grain Servings: 1
- Protein Servings: 1
- Fruit Servings: ½
- Vegetable Servings: ½

Ingredients:

Grain Component:

- 1 oz. dry old-fashioned oats

Protein Component:

- 1 oz. chopped pecans
- 4 oz. yogurt

Fruit/Vegetable Component:

- 3 oz. pumpkin puree
- 3 oz. sliced banana or blueberries

Other Ingredients:

- 1-2 tsp. pumpkin pie spice
- Alternatively, combine 1/8 tsp. each cinnamon, fresh ground nutmeg, and cloves

Additions for Those on Maintenance Plans:

- *Grain Component:* Increase oats to 1 ½ oz.
- *Protein Component:* Increase pecans, yogurt, or add hemp, flax, chia seeds.
- *Fat Component:* Add more nuts or nut butter.

Directions:

1. Combine oats and pumpkin pie spice.

2. Combine oats with the amount of water specified on the package. Cook oats in a medium sauce pan on the stove top according to package directions.

3. After the oats have finished cooking, and while they're still warm, stir in the pumpkin puree.

4. Stir in the fruit, nuts, and yogurt.

Not Really Quiche

Number of Servings: Makes 3 Servings

Time Required: About 60 minutes

Components of Each Serving:

- Grain Servings: 1
- Protein Servings: 1
- Vegetable Servings: 1

Ingredients:

Grain Component:

- 12 oz. potatoes or sweet potatoes

Protein Component:

- 5 eggs, beaten
- 4 oz. low-fat or skim milk

Vegetable Component: (Use these ingredients in any combination to make up the appropriate weight for a vegetable serving.)

- Asparagus
- Tomatoes
- Mushrooms
- Broccoli
- Peppers
- Spinach or kale
- Onions
- Artichoke hearts

Other Ingredients:

- Salt, pepper, and nutmeg to taste
- Chives or green onions, chopped, to garnish

Additions for Those on Maintenance Plans:

- *Grain Component:* Add cooked quinoa to the filling mixture.
- *Protein Component:* Add small amount of breakfast sausage to the filling mixture.
- *Fat Component:* Garnish with avocado.

Directions:

1. Preheat the oven to 400 degrees Fahrenheit.
2. Peel and slice the potatoes or sweet potatoes into ¼-inch-thick slices
3. Lightly oil a casserole dish with a small amount of oil, then place the potatoes in a single layer on the bottom of the dish.
4. Season the potatoes with salt and pepper.
5. Bake for about 15 minutes, just until the potatoes are beginning to brown.
6. While the potatoes cook, prepare and weigh the vegetables.
7. In a medium mixing bowl, whisk the milk together with the eggs until the eggs are well beaten. Season with salt, pepper and nutmeg.
8. Remove the casserole dish from the oven and reduce the heat to 375 degrees.
9. Layer the vegetables over the potatoes in the dish, then pour the egg mixture over the vegetables.
10. Season again with salt and pepper, and then place the dish back in the oven.
11. Bake until the egg is completely set in the center. This should take about 45 minutes.
12. Garnish with chives or green onions.

Salads and Dressings

The main ingredients in most salads--vegetables and fruits--aren't subject to any strict prohibitions in the Bright Line Eating plan, so salads can and should make up a large part of a Bright Line diet. They give you the opportunity to combine diverse ingredients in interesting and satisfying ways, and they also help to ensure that you're eating a balanced diet even within the confines of the Bright Line structure.

You could stick with simple, traditional salads by combining a serving of fresh greens and other salad veggies with a reasonable amount of Bright-Line-compliant dressing. But we know that eating one basic salad after another can get very boring, so we've collected the most interesting salad recipes we could find. These recipes draw upon unexpected ingredients and seasonings, and they combine those ingredients in often unusual ways.

We've also focused on recipes that include grains and proteins, so if you want to build your diet solely around salads for a while, you can do just that without worrying that you're not getting balanced nutrition.

Most of these recipes take their proteins from non-meat sources, but we've included one savory salad that's right at home at any backyard barbecue.

And we've included a few recipes for Bright-Line-friendly salad dressings, too, so you'll always be prepared to turn any garden harvest into a meal that fits perfectly within your diet plan.

Black Bean Fruit Salad

Number of Servings: Makes 2 Servings

Time Required: About 60 minutes

Components of Each Serving:

- Protein Servings: 1
- Vegetable Servings: 1
- Fat Servings: 1
- Fruit Servings: 1
- Grain Servings: 1

Ingredients:

Vegetable Component:

- 1 red pepper
- 1 red onion
- Salad greens to reach vegetable serving total weight

Protein Component:

- 12 oz. canned black beans

Fruit Component:

- 1 large ripe mango or peach

Fat Component:

- 1 avocado (2 fat servings)

Grain Component:

- 8 oz. cooked brown rice (approx. ½ cup dry)

Other Ingredients:

- 2 cloves garlic, minced
- ½ tsp. cumin

Ingredients for dressing:

- Juice of 1 small lime
- Fresh cilantro, chopped
- 1 tablespoon white vinegar
- Pinch of salt
- 1 clove garlic

Directions:

1. Prepare the rice according to directions on the package.
2. While rice is cooking, heat a skillet over medium heat. Sauté the onions and red peppers with a dash of oil, just until they begin to soften, about 5 minutes.
3. Weigh the black beans and add to the skillet along with the cumin and garlic. Add salt and pepper to taste.
4. Put the dressing ingredients in a blender or food processor and pulse to combine.
5. Peel and dice the mango (or peach).
6. Weigh rice and add to a salad bowl.
7. Weigh salad greens and lay them on top of the rice.
8. Add bean mixture on top of greens, and top the whole thing with diced mango and dressing.

Marinated Mushroom Salad

Number of Servings: Makes 1 Serving
Time Required: About 60 minutes

Components of Each Serving:

- Protein Servings: 1
- Vegetable Servings: 1
- Fat Servings: 1

Ingredients:

Vegetable Component:

- 1 large portobello mushroom

The remainder of a vegetable serving's weight should come from a combination of these ingredients:

- Salad greens
- Tomatoes
- Red onions

Protein Component:

- 3 oz. canned chickpeas, rinsed and drained
- 1 oz nuts or seeds (walnuts, sunflower seeds, pine nuts, or other nuts)

Fat Component:

(dressing for 1 serving)

- 1 Tbsp. grapeseed oil (or sub olive or canola oil)
- 1 Tbsp. red wine vinegar
- 1 Tbsp. spicy, smooth mustard

(1 serving of marinade for the mushroom):

- 2 tsp. olive oil
- 1 Tbsp. soy sauce
- 1 Tbsp. balsamic vinegar
- 1 clove garlic

Other Ingredients:

- 1-2 tsp. vanilla extract
- 1 tsp. ground cinnamon
- 1/8 tsp. nutmeg
- ¼ tsp. salt

Additions for Those on Maintenance Plans:

- *Grain Component:* Add 4 oz. of cooked quinoa.
- *Protein Component:* Increase total amount of nuts or add beans.
- *Fat Component:* Add chopped fresh avocado.

Directions:

1. Preheat the oven to 400 degrees Fahrenheit.
2. Combine all marinade ingredients in a small mixing bowl.
3. Place the mushroom upside down, with the bottom of the cap facing up, in an oven safe dish. Pour the marinade into each mushroom cap. Allow to marinate at room temperature for about 20 minutes.
4. Cover the baking dish with aluminum foil and place in the oven. Roast for 30 minutes.
5. Remove the foil, turn the mushroom over. Cook, uncovered, for another 10 minutes.
6. Mix the dressing ingredients in a small mixing bowl.
7. Remove the mushroom from the oven when it is done, and allow it to cool let it cool for about 5 minutes. Slice into ½-inch-thick slices.
8. Weigh the mushroom for each serving, then add salad ingredients to reach appropriate total weight for the vegetable serving. Add protein ingredients, followed by the dressing.

Beet and Fruit Salad

Number of Servings: Makes 2 Servings

Time Required: About 90 minutes

Components of Each Serving:

- Vegetable Servings: 1
- Protein Servings: 1
- Fat Servings: 1
- Fruit Servings: 1

Ingredients:

Vegetable Component:

- 2 bunches of beets
- Salad greens (lettuce, arugula, shredded cabbage, kale, etc.) to make up vegetable serving weight

Protein and Fat Servings:

These ingredients are used to make a pesto (2 proteins + 2 fats):

- 4 oz. pine nuts or walnuts (2 protein servings)
- 1 oz. olive oil (2 fat servings)
- 1 bunch cilantro
- 2 cloves garlic
- ½ large lime (or 1 small lime)
- Pinch of salt

Fruit Serving:

- 2 oranges

Additions for Those on Maintenance Plans:

- *Grain Additions:* Add 4 oz. of cooked quinoa.

- *Protein Additions:* Add more nuts or chickpeas.
- *Fat Additions:* Add chopped fresh avocado.

Directions:

1. Cut the stems off the beets and boil them whole, unpeeled, in a large pot of water. Keep the lid on as they boil for about 1 hour.
2. When the beets are tender, drain them and allow them to cool. Then run them under cold water; the peels should slip off easily.
3. Dice the beets.
4. Peel the oranges and separate them into wedges if you prefer.
5. Place all the pesto ingredients into a food processor or blender and pulse to combine.
6. Weigh the beets and salad greens to make up a vegetable serving. Top with orange wedges.
7. Divide the pesto into 2 equal portions, and top the salad with one portion.

Quinoa Green Salad

Number of Servings: Makes 1 Serving

Time Required: About 15 minutes

Components of Each Serving:

- Vegetable Servings: 1
- Protein Servings: 1
- Fat Servings: 1

Ingredients:

Vegetable Component: (Use a combination of these and other salad veggies to make up a vegetable serving total weight.)

- Cherry tomatoes, halved
- Red bell pepper, diced
- Kale, roughly chopped

Protein Component:

Include any two of these ingredients:

- 2 oz. cooked quinoa
- 3 oz. canned chickpeas or black beans
- 1 oz. walnuts or other nuts

Fat and Protein Component:

- ½ oz. olive oil

(For dressing):

- 3 oz. avocado (about ½ of a large avocado)
- 6 oz. low-fat or skim milk
- 1-2 Tbsp. lemon juice
- 1 ½ tsp. white wine vinegar
- 1-2 cloves garlic

- ¼ tsp. dried dill
- ½ tsp. dried parsley
- ½ tsp. onion powder
- Salt to taste

Other Ingredients:
- 2 tsp. fresh lemon juice

Additions for Those on Maintenance Plans:
- *Grain Additions:* Add 4 oz. roasted potatoes.
- *Protein Additions:* Add a third protein from the list of protein ingredients.
- *Fat Additions:* Add chopped fresh avocado.

Directions:
Toss everything together and enjoy!

Avocado Salad

Number of Servings: Makes 1 Serving
Time Required: About 15 minutes

Components of Each Serving:

- Vegetable Servings: 1
- Protein Servings: 1
- Fat Servings: 1

Ingredients:

Vegetable Component: (Use these vegetables in combination to make up the right total vegetable weight.)

- Romaine lettuce, chopped
- Corn
- Cherry tomatoes, halved
- Bell peppers, diced
- Cucumbers, diced
- Carrots, shredded
- Green onions, chopped

Protein Serving:

- 1 serving avocado ranch dressing (contains ¼ protein)
- 4 oz. chickpeas (¾ protein)

Fat Serving:

- 2 ½ oz. avocado ranch dressing (contains ½ fat)
- 1 oz. fresh avocado

Other Ingredients:

- Sugar-free barbecue sauce

Additions for Those on Maintenance Plans:

- *Grain Additions:* Add 4 oz. cooked quinoa.
- *Protein Additions:* Add walnuts.
- *Fat Additions:* Add more fresh avocado.

Directions:

1. Combine all the dressing ingredients in a blender or food processor and pulse to thoroughly puree and combine.
2. In a saucepan, combine chickpeas and barbecue sauce and simmer over medium-low heat for about 10 minutes.
3. Prepare and weigh vegetable and toss with dressing.
4. Place salad greens on a serving plate and top with still-warm barbecue chickpeas.

Thai Salad

Number of Servings: Makes 2 Servings

Time Required: About 20 minutes

Components of Each Serving:

- Protein Servings: 1
- Fat Servings: 1
- Vegetable Servings: 1

Ingredients:

Vegetable Component: (Weigh out enough of these ingredients to make two vegetable servings.)

- Shredded cabbage
- Kale, chopped
- Carrots, shredded or grated
- Cucumber, peeled and chopped
- Red bell pepper, seeded and chopped

Protein Component:

- 2 eggs

Grain Component:

- 1 oz. dry quinoa (makes 4 oz. cooked)
- 4 oz. edamame, shelled and cooked

Other Ingredients:

- 1 oz. peanut butter
- 1 tsp. grated fresh ginger
- 1 tsp. soy sauce or tamari
- 1 tsp. rice vinegar

- Dash of hot pepper sauce
- Juice of ½ lime

Additions for Those on Maintenance Plans:

- *Grain Component:* Increase dry quinoa amount to 1 ½ oz.
- *Protein Component:* Increase edamame or add peanuts as a topping.
- *Fat Component:* Add a teaspoon sesame oil to the quinoa.

Directions:

1. Cook quinoa according to package directions and allow to cool.
2. In a medium mixing bowl, add the other ingredients, excluding the edamame, and stir together. Add a little water as necessary to make the dressing into the desired consistency.
3. Toss the quinoa and edamame with the dressing. Serve garnished with chopped fresh cilantro or basil.

BBQ Pork and Cabbage Salad

Number of Servings: Makes 4 Servings
Time Required: About 3 hours

Components of Each Serving:
- Protein Servings: 1
- Fat Servings: 1
- Vegetable Servings: 1

Ingredients:
Vegetable Component:
- Cabbage, chopped
- Carrots, shredded

Fat and Protein Component:
- 1 lb. bone-in pork ribs
- ½ tsp. paprika
- 1 tsp. garlic salt

(For dressing):
- 1 tsp. mayonnaise
- ½ tsp. apple cider vinegar
- ½ tsp. fresh lime juice

Other Ingredients:
- Salt and pepper to taste

Directions:
1. Preheat oven to 325 degrees Fahrenheit.
2. Combine garlic salt, paprika, salt and pepper in a small bowl. Rub the mixture thoroughly over both sides of the pork ribs.

3. Wrap ribs loosely in aluminum foil and place on a baking sheet. Put the sheet in the oven and roast the ribs until tender, about 2 ½ to 3 hours.
4. Weigh a combination of the vegetables to make up a vegetable serving.
5. In a small bowl, whisk together mayonnaise, vinegar and lime juice. Toss the dressing with the vegetables.
6. When the ribs are finished cooking, allow them to cool for 15 minutes, then remove them carefully from the bones, shredding the meat with your fingers.
7. Top the salad on a serving plate with 4 ounces of the shredded meat.

Bright Ranch Dressing

Number of Servings: Makes 3 Servings

Time Required: About 15 minutes

Components of Each Serving:

- Protein Servings: ¼
- Fat Servings: ½

Ingredients:

Protein Component:

- 6 oz. low-fat or skim milk

Fat Component:

- 3 oz. avocado (about ½ of a large avocado)

Other ingredients:

- 1-2 Tbsp. fresh lemon juice, adjusting to taste
- 1 ½ tsp. white wine vinegar
- 1-2 cloves garlic, chopped
- ¼ tsp. dried dill
- ½ tsp. dried parsley
- ½ tsp. onion powder
- Salt to taste

Directions:

1. Combine all the ingredients in a blender or food processor. Blend until the mixture is smooth.
2. The dressing can be stored in a sealed container in the refrigerator for up to 3 days.

Bright Caesar Dressing

Number of Servings: Makes 2 Servings

Time Required: About 15 minutes

Components of Each Serving:

- Protein Servings: ½

Ingredients:

Protein Component:

- 4 oz. plain hummus

Other ingredients:

- 1 tsp. dijon mustard
- ½ tsp. lemon zest
- 2 Tbsp. fresh lemon juice, adjusting to taste
- 2 tsp. capers
- 3 tsp. pickle juice
- 4-5 cloves garlic, minced

Directions:

1. Combine all the ingredients in a blender or food processor. Blend until the mixture is smooth. Add water if necessary to achieve the desired consistency.
2. The dressing can be stored in a sealed container in the refrigerator for up to 3 days.

Bright Goddess Dressing

Number of Servings: Makes 4 Servings

Time Required: About 15 minutes

Components of Each Serving:

- Protein Servings: ¼
- Fat Servings: 1

Ingredients:

Protein Component:

- 2 oz. pistachios, shelled

Fat Component:

- 2 oz. fresh avocado
- 3 Tbsp. olive oil

Other ingredients:

- 1 cup fresh parsley
- ½ small jalapeño pepper, seeded and chopped
- 1 clove garlic, chopped
- Juice of 1-2 limes, adjusting to taste
- ½ tsp. salt

Directions:

1. Combine all the ingredients in a blender or food processor. Blend until the mixture is smooth. Add water if necessary to achieve the desired consistency.
2. The dressing can be stored in a sealed container in the refrigerator for up to 3 days.

Bright Pesto

Number of Servings: Makes 2 Servings

Time Required: About 15 minutes

Components of Each Serving:

- Protein Servings: 1
- Fat Servings: 1

Ingredients:

Protein Component:

- 4 oz. walnuts, chopped

Fat Component:

- 2 Tbsp. olive oil

Other ingredients:

- 2 cups (pack) fresh basil leaves
- Juice of 1 lemon
- 3 cloves garlic, chopped
- ½ tsp. salt

Directions:

1. Combine all the ingredients in a blender or food processor. Pulse to chop all the ingredients, and then blend continuously until the mixture is only slightly chunky.
2. The dressing can be stored in a sealed container in the refrigerator for 1-2 days.

Soups

Is there a better kind of food than soup? A warm soup is as comforting as can be on a chilly day, and settling down with a hearty soup when the weather is bad is the very definition of comfort food. But soups can also bring the freshness and bright flavors of spring and summer into your home, as they incorporate ingredients that take advantage of the bounty of the growing season.

The best soup recipes have an appeal beyond their delicious ingredients, too. The best soup recipes are very easy to make; just through some ingredients into a pot and allow their flavors to meld into something wonderful. When you're busy and hungry, and you need an easy meal that doesn't ask too much of you, a simple soup more often than not is just what you're looking for.

We've collected soup recipes here that explore the full spectrum of soup possibilities. We've included simple soups that rely on the strong character of their ingredients and come together in a matter of minutes. We've also included more complex soups that take a little more time and effort to craft, but that are well worth it. And we've even included some fix-it-and-forget-it soups that make your slow cooker do all the work while you get more important things done.

We've also tried to give you some options in terms of serving options. Traditional soups are often concocted in giant pots and deliver enough sustenance for an army. That's great if you have an army to feed, but if you're trying to follow a precise Bright Line Eating plan and are just trying to feed yourself, the quantities can be overwhelming. So we've included soup recipes that are more tightly focused on satisfying your plan requirements. Some of them produce just a few servings, so you can use them in a single meal for yourself and your family. Others produce a little more, so you can divide them and use them for a handful of meals through the week. Either way, we're giving you the tools to make fantastic soups on a scale that's right for you and your plan.

Squash Soup

Number of Servings: Makes 6 Servings

Time Required: About 90 minutes

Components of Each Serving:
- Protein Servings: 1
- Fat Servings: 1
- Vegetable Servings: 1

Ingredients:

Vegetable Component: (Weigh out enough of these ingredients * to make six vegetable servings.)
- 1 butternut squash, peeled with and seeded*
- 1 medium sweet onion, chopped*
- 1 small bag of baby carrots*
- 2 cans (15 oz. each) vegetable broth

Protein Component:
- 1 cup low-fat or skim milk

Fat Component:
- 4 Tbsp. butter

Other Ingredients:
- Garlic salt
- Italian spice mix

Directions:
1. Preheat oven to 350 degrees Fahrenheit.
2. Chop butternut squash, onion, and carrots into bite-size pieces.

3. Toss vegetables with a dash of olive oil and sprinkle with garlic salt and Italian spices.

4. Place into a baking dishes and put onto the center rack of the oven.

5. Roast until they're fork tender. This should take about 50-60 minutes.

6. Place roasted vegetables into a food processor or blender. Add about 3 cups vegetable broth. Blend until the mixture is a smooth puree, adding more broth if necessary to reach the desired consistency.

7. Add puree to a large pot with 1 cup of milk and 4 tablespoons butter. Heat on medium-low heat, stirring constantly, until butter is melted and the soup is hot.

8. Season to taste with salt, pepper and more garlic seasoning if desired.

Squash and Bean Soup

Number of Servings: Makes 3 Servings

Time Required: About 90 minutes

Components of Each Serving:

- Protein Servings: 1
- Fat Servings: 1
- Vegetable Servings: 1

Ingredients:

Vegetable Component:

- 1 acorn squash, seeded
- ½ yellow onion, diced
- ½ red bell pepper, diced
- ½ lb. shiitake mushrooms, sliced

Protein Component:

- 18 oz. adzuki beans

Fat Component:

- 1 ½ Tbsp. olive oil
- 1 ½ Tbsp. sesame oil

Other Ingredients:

- 2 cups vegetable broth
- 1 clove garlic, minced
- 1 tsp. fresh ginger, peeled and grated
- 1 tsp. Chinese five-spice powder
- ¼ tsp. salt
- 2 tsp. fresh lime juice
- ¼ tsp. soy sauce

Directions:

1. Preheat the oven to 400 degrees Fahrenheit. Cut the acorn squash in half, scoop out the seeds with a spoon, and roast face down on a baking sheet lined with parchment paper.

2. Roast the squash until it's soft. This should take 30-45 minutes. Remove the squash from the oven and allow to cool slightly, then use a spoon to scoop the flesh from the squash shell.

3. Sauté the onions and peppers in 1 ½ tablespoon olive oil in a skillet over medium-high heat. Saute just until the onion begins to brown, which should be about 7-10 minutes.

4. Combine the squash, onions and peppers and weigh them to reach a total of three 6-ounce servings (or the appropriate weight for three of your plan's vegetable servings).

5. Put the weighed vegetables in a medium stock pot.

6. Add the ginger and garlic and sauté for 1 more minute over medium heat, just until the ginger and garlic are fragrant.

7. Add the salt and five-spice, and cook for another minute, again until the spices become fragrant. Add the vegetable stock.

8. Cover the pot and bring to a boil.

9. Lower the heat and simmer for about 10-15 more minutes.

10. Weigh out three 6-ounce servings of the adzuki beans. Add them and the lime juice to the pot.

11. Cover and reduce the heat to low. Simmer over low heat until the beans are heated, about 5 minutes.

12. In a skillet, heat the 1 ½ tablespoons of sesame oil over medium heat.

13. Brown the mushrooms in the skillet, about 7 minutes.

14. Add ¼ teaspoon soy sauce and stir for about another minute.

15. Divide the warm soup into 3 equal servings in serving bowls. Top each bowl with a third of the mushrooms.

Veggie Chili

Servings: Makes 4 Servings

Time Required: About 6-8 hours

Components of Each Serving:

- Vegetable Serving: 1
- Protein Serving: 1
- Fat Serving: 1

Ingredients:

Vegetable Component:

- 1 medium onion, chopped
- 1 medium bell pepper, chopped
- 3-4 carrots, chopped
- 1 can (15 oz.) pumpkin puree
- 1 can (14.5 oz.) diced tomatoes

Protein Component:

- 3 cans (15 oz. each) black beans, rinsed and drained

Fat Component:

- 8 oz. fresh chopped avocado

Other Ingredients:

- 2 tsp. smoked paprika
- 3 tsp. chili powder
- 2 tsp. dried oregano
- 1 tsp. cumin
- 3 garlic cloves, minced
- 1 cup vegetable broth

Additions for Those on Maintenance Plans:

- *Grain Additions:* Serve over rice.
- *Protein Additions:* Increase the amount of beans.
- *Fat Additions:* Increase the amount of avocado.

Directions:

1. Put all ingredients, excluding the avocado, into a slow cooker.
2. Cook on the slow cooker's low setting for 6-8 hours.
3. Divide equally into 4 servings.
4. Serve topped with 2 ounces of sliced avocado.

Thai-Style Yellow Curry

Servings: Makes 4 Servings

Time Required: About 30 minutes

Components of Each Serving:

- Veggie Serving: 1
- Protein Serving: 1
- Fat Serving: 1
- Fruit Serving: ½

Ingredients:

Vegetable Component: (Combine these ingredients to make the appropriate weight for 4 vegetable servings.)

- 1 medium onion
- 1 red bell pepper
- 1 large head of broccoli
- Frozen peas

Protein Component:

- 8 oz. roasted whole cashews

Fat Component:

- 10 oz. regular fat coconut milk

Fruit Component:

- 2 fresh mangos, diced

Other Ingredients:

- 2 Tbsp. minced fresh ginger
- 2 Tbsp. minced garlic
- ½ tsp. chili paste

- 1-3 tsp. red curry paste
- 2-3 tsp. soy sauce
- 2 tsp. ground turmeric
- Pinch of salt
- Juice of 1 lemon
- Fresh basil or cilantro, chopped

Additions for Those on Maintenance Plans:
- *Grain Additions:* Serve over 4 oz cooked rice or quinoa.
- *Protein Additions:* Add more cashews.
- *Fat Additions:* Increase coconut milk or cashews.

Directions:
1. Chop and weigh the onion, red pepper, broccoli, and peas to reach the desired weight.
2. Peel and grate the ginger and garlic.
3. In a heavy bottomed pot over medium heat, sauté the onion, ginger, garlic, chili paste, and curry paste in a dash of coconut oil, until fragrant and softened. This should take only 1-2 minutes.
4. Add coconut milk, salt, soy sauce, and turmeric, then simmer over medium heat for 7-10 minutes.
5. Add all the vegetables, excluding the peas, to the pot.
6. Cover and simmer for 5-10 minutes, stirring occasionally.
7. Add mangoes, peas, and lemon juice and stir to combine. Simmer over low heat for 3-4 minutes.
8. Garnish with cashews and fresh basil or cilantro.

Thai-Style Chickpea Curry

Servings: Makes 3 Servings

Time Required: About 30 minutes

Components of Each Serving:

- Vegetable Serving: 1
- Protein Serving: 1
- Fat Serving: 1

Ingredients:

Vegetable Component:

- 1 medium yellow onion, chopped
- 2-3 carrots, peeled and chopped
- 1 can (15 oz.) diced tomatoes
- 1 can (15 oz.) pumpkin puree

Protein Component:

- 18 oz. canned chickpeas, rinsed and drained

Fat Component:

- 12 oz. light coconut milk

Other Ingredients:

- 1-2 Tbsp. curry powder
- ½ tsp. salt
- ¼ tsp. black pepper
- ¼ tsp. turmeric
- ¼ tsp. cinnamon
- 1/8 tsp. cayenne pepper
- 2 garlic cloves, minced

- ½-inch piece of fresh ginger, peeled and minced
- 1 cup water
- ½ lime or lemon

Additions for Those on Maintenance Plans:
- *Grain Additions:* Serve over 4 ounces rice or quinoa.
- *Protein Additions:* Add more chickpeas.
- *Fat Additions:* Add more coconut milk.

Directions:
1. In a large pot over medium heat, sweat the carrots and the onion, covered, for 3-5 minutes, just until onion begins to soften.
2. Add garlic and ginger and cook for 1 more minute, until the garlic is fragrant.
3. Add the tomatoes, pumpkin, chickpeas, curry powder, ginger, salt, pepper, turmeric, cinnamon, and cayenne pepper. Stir to combined. Reduce heat to low and simmer for 10 minutes.
4. Pour the coconut milk and water into the pot, stirring to combine thoroughly.
5. Simmer gently over low heat for 15-20 minutes, until the carrots are tender when pierced with the tip of a knife. Bringing the curry to a boil may curdle the coconut milk, so take care not to get it too hot.
6. When the carrots are finished cooking, stir in the lemon juice and season to taste with salt and pepper.

Spicy Peanut Soup

Servings: Makes 4 Servings

Time Required: About 40 minutes

Components of Each Serving:

- Vegetable Serving: 1
- Protein Serving: 1
- Fat Serving: 1

Ingredients:

Vegetable Component:

- 3-4 fresh jalapeños, seeded and minced (or 1 bell pepper, seeded and chopped, if you'd like to tone down the spice)
- 8 oz. fresh spinach, stemmed and chopped
- 1 large onion, diced
- 2 cans (14 oz. each) diced tomatoes in juice
- 2 large carrots, sliced

Protein Component:

- 8 oz. smooth natural peanut butter

Fat Component:

- 8 oz. light coconut milk
- 2 Tbsp. vegetable oil

Other Ingredients:

- Cayenne pepper, adjusting for spice preferences
- 2 Tbsp. curry powder
- 3 cups vegetable stock
- 1-2 garlic cloves, minced

- ¼ cup chopped fresh cilantro
- Salt and pepper, to taste

Additions for Those on Maintenance Plans:
- *Grain Additions:* Serve over 4 oz. cooked rice or quinoa.
- *Protein Additions:* Add more peanut butter.
- *Fat Additions:* Add more peanut butter.

Directions:
1. In a large pot, heat the oil over medium-high heat. Add the onion, garlic, jalapeños or bell pepper and cilantro. Cook about 10-12 minutes, just until the onion has is beginning to brown.
2. Add the carrots, cayenne and curry powder. Saute until the spices become fragrant, about one minute more.
3. Add the stock and tomatoes with the juices from the can. Stir thoroughly and bring to a boil.
4. Reduce the heat to low and simmer gently, stirring frequently, until the carrots are tender, about 20 minutes.
5. Add the peanut butter, coconut milk and spinach. Cook until the spinach has wilted and the soup begins to thicken, about 10 minutes more.
6. Season with salt and pepper to taste.

Pumpkin Soup

Servings: Makes 4 Servings

Time Required: About 30 minutes

Components of Each Serving:

- Vegetable Serving: 1
- Protein Serving: 1

Ingredients:

Vegetable Component:

- 1 ½ cans pumpkin puree
- 3 cups vegetable broth
- 1 large yellow onion

Protein Component:

- 1 cup low-fat or skim milk

Other Ingredients:

- 1 tsp. garlic salt
- 2 Tbsp. pumpkin pie spice

Directions:

1. Peel and finely chop the onion.
2. Combine the onion, pumpkin puree, broth, milk, garlic salt, and pumpkin pie spice in a large pot.
3. Bring the mixture to a boil, then reduce heat to low. Simmer just until the soup begins to think, about 10-15 minutes.
4. Allow the soup to cool for about 15 minutes.
5. Carefully transfer the soup to a blender, and blend until it has a smooth consistency.
6. Season to taste with salt and pepper.

Corn Chowder

Servings: Makes 4 Servings

Time Required: About 45 minutes

Components of Each Serving:

- Vegetable Serving: 1
- Protein Serving: 1
- Fat Serving: 1
- Grain Serving: 1

Ingredients:

Vegetable Component: (Use a combination of these ingredients to total the appropriate weight for 4 vegetable servings.)

- Carrots, diced
- Corn (fresh or frozen)
- Onion, diced
- Celery, diced
- Red pepper, diced
- Chopped kale

Protein Component: (Use only one of the following protein options.)

- 24 oz. white beans
- 16 oz. veggie sausage
- Or a combination of 12 oz. white beans and 8 oz. veggie sausage

Fat Component:

Use only one of the following fat options:

- 2 oz. cooking oil
- 4 oz. regular fat coconut milk

Grain Component:

- 2 large yellow potatoes, peeled and diced

Other Ingredients:

- 2 cloves garlic, minced
- 4 cups vegetable broth
- ½ tsp. dried dill
- ½ tsp. salt
- Ground black pepper to taste

Directions:

1. Prepare the vegetables by peeling, dicing and weighing them.
2. Add either oil (if that's the fat option you've chosen) or ¼ cup water to the pot.
3. Heat the pot over medium-high heat.
4. Add the garlic to the pot and saute, until the garlic is fragrant but not browned and the vegetables are beginning to brown, about 10 minutes
5. Add the vegetable broth, potatoes, and spices.
6. Bring to a boil, and then reduce heat to low and cover the pot. Simmer for 15-20 minutes, just until potatoes are fork tender.
7. Add the beans and/or veggie sausage, corn, and kale. Stir thoroughly and simmer until everything is heated, about 5 minutes.
8. Remove the pot from the heat and stir in the coconut milk, if you've chosen it as your fat option.

Mushroom Soup

Servings: Makes 4 Servings

Time Required: About 90 minutes

Components of Each Serving:

- Vegetable Serving: 1
- Protein Serving: 1
- Fat Serving: 1
- Grain Serving: 1

Ingredients:

Vegetable Component:

- 1 lb. fresh mushrooms, chopped
- 1 small onion, diced
- 2-3 medium carrots, diced
- 2-3 celery stalks, diced

Protein Component:

- 3 oz. cashews
- 1 can (15 oz.) white beans

Grain Component:

- 4 oz. dried pearl barley

Fat Component:

- 4 Tbsp. olive oil

Other Ingredients:

- 4 cloves garlic cloves, minced
- 2 tsp. dried thyme
- 7 cups low sodium vegetable broth, divided
- 1 ½ Tbsp. soy sauce

Directions:

1. Heat 2 tablespoons oil in a large, heavy-bottomed pot over medium-high heat.

2. When the oil is hot, add the mushrooms. Saute until the mushrooms are browned, about 10 minutes.

3. Add the remainder of the oil, onion, carrot, celery, and garlic, and saut--é until vegetables are beginning to soften, about 5 minutes.

4. Add 1 cup broth and thyme to the pot. Allow the soup to come to a boil, then reduce the heat to low and bring the soup down to a simmer. Simmer until the soup is reduced by half, about 5-10 minutes.

5. Add 5 more cups of broth and the barley to the pot. Increase the heat and bring the soup to a boil again.

6. Lower heat the heat once more to bring the soup back to a simmer. Simmer, uncovered, until the barley is tender, about 45 minutes.

7. Carefully transfer 1 cup of the soup to a blender. Add another cup of vegetable stock and the cashews to the blender. Blend until the mixture is smooth, and then return it to the pot.

8. Add the beans the beans to the pot.

9. Stir thoroughly to ensure that all the ingredients are well combined, and continue to simmer until everything is heated through.

10. Divide into 4 equal servings.

Lentil Soup

Servings: Makes 6 Servings

Time Required: About 75 minutes

Components of Each Serving:

- Vegetable Serving: 1
- Protein Serving: 1
- Fat Serving: 1

Ingredients:

Vegetable Component:

- Onion, diced
- Carrots, chopped
- 2 cans (28 oz. each) diced tomatoes, with juice
- 2 cups chopped fresh kale

Protein Component:

- 2 cups dry brown, green, or yellow large lentils, rinsed

Fat Component:

- 6 Tbsp. olive oil

Other Ingredients:

- 8 cups vegetable broth
- 4 cups water
- 2 tsp. salt
- Red pepper flakes, to taste
- Freshly ground black pepper
- 6 cloves garlic, minced
- 4 tsp. ground cumin

- 2 tsp. curry powder
- 1 tsp. dried thyme
- Juice of ½ lemon

Additions for Those on Maintenance Plans:
- *Grain Additions:* Serve over 4 oz. cooked rice or quinoa.
- *Protein Additions:* Increase amount of lentils.
- *Fat Additions:* Top with chopped fresh avocado.

Directions:
1. Heat the olive oil over medium-high heat in a large, heavy-bottomed stock pot or dutch oven.
2. Add the chopped onion and carrot to the pot. Saute just until vegetables are beginning to soften, about 5 minutes.
3. Add the garlic, cumin, curry powder and thyme. Cook until fragrant, stirring constantly, about 1 minutes.
4. Add the canned tomatoes with their juice. Cook, stirring, for about 5 minutes.
5. Add the lentils, broth and water.
6. Add salt, freshly ground black pepper, and a dash of red pepper flakes.
7. Increase heat to bring the soup to a boil, then reduce heat to low to bring the pot down to a simmer.
8. Cook, uncovered, until the lentils are tender but not yet beginning to break down. This should take about 30 minutes.
9. Remove the pot from heat and stir in lemon juice. Season to taste with more salt and pepper if necessary.
10. Add kale while the soup is hot and stir until the greens are wilted.
11. Divide into 6 equal servings and serve hot.

Main Dishes and Sides

Soups and salads are a delicious and essential part of every meal plan. There's no question about that. But sometimes you want something more substantial to build your meal around. To keep you happy at those times, we've included these main dish and side dish recipes. When you need a truly hearty meal, this is the section to turn to.

Here we've collected recipes that are creative and surprising. They don't just grudgingly adhere to the restrictions of the Bright Line Eating plan; they fully embrace the restrictions as an opportunity to try new ingredients and look for different sources of nutrients than the conventional Western diet is built upon.

To that end, many of the recipes look beyond the prohibited processed flour for new sources of fiber and other nutrients found in grains. Many of them include quinoa and rice, and other pull in the wonderful texture and flavor of polenta to build savory dishes that will satisfy the most robust hunger and give you the nutrients that you need.

And if you're more concerned with the absence of the fun from ingredients like pasta, we've included recipes that use innovative solutions to replace what's missing. Spend some time with spaghetti squash, and you might find that you don't miss real spaghetti at all.

Many of the recipes also incorporate alternative sources of protein, so if you want to use them as replacements for meat in your diet, they're up to the task. Chickpeas, nuts, eggs, tofu and mushrooms all make appearances, and they're used in delightful ways.

We've emphasized, in these recipes, the use of fresh ingredients when we can, because we believe that even if your meal plans are regimented, they should still be delicious and nutritious.

Most of these recipes are interesting and filling enough to be the centerpiece of a meal all on their own, but they can play a supporting role, as well. Pair them with your favorite meat dishes or use them in combination to fill out the structure of each of your meals, and you can't go wrong.

Spicy Quinoa Skillet

Number of Servings: Makes 4 Servings

Time Required: About 40 minutes

Components of Each Serving:

- Protein Servings: 1
- Fat Servings: 1
- Vegetable Servings: 1

Ingredients:

Vegetable Component:

- 1 can fire-roasted diced tomatoes, with liquid
- 1 cup corn, frozen or canned
- 1 small onion, diced
- 1 bell pepper, diced
- 1 jalapeño, seeded and chopped

Protein Component:

- 2 eggs

Grain Component:

- 4 oz. dry quinoa (makes 16 oz. cooked)

Fat Component:

- 1 Tbsp. olive oil

Other Ingredients:

- 2 Tbsp. fresh cilantro, chopped
- 1 tsp. chili powder
- ½ tsp. cumin
- Salt and pepper, to taste

- 2 cloves garlic, minced
- 1 cup vegetable broth

Directions:

1. Heat olive oil in a large skillet over medium-high heat.
2. Add onion and pepper until soft and the onion is translucent. It should take about 5 minutes.
3. Add garlic and jalapeño pepper. Saute, stirring frequently, about 1 minute, just until the pepper is fragrant.
4. Stir in quinoa, and the remaining ingredients.
5. Bring mixture to a boil, then cover and reduce the heat to low.
6. Simmer, covered but stirring occasionally, until the quinoa is cooked through. This should take about 20 minutes. If all the broth is absorbed before the quinoa is cooked, add a little water.
7. Season with salt and pepper and divide into four equal servings.

Sweet Potatoes and Lentils

Number of Servings: Makes 3 Servings

Time Required: About 60 minutes

Components of Each Serving:

- Protein Servings: 1
- Fat Servings: 1
- Grain Servings: 1
- Vegetable Servings: 1

Ingredients:

Vegetable Component: (Weigh a mixture of these vegetables to equal three servings.)

- 1 bunch kale, spinach or other salad greens
- 1 bunch asparagus
- 1 red pepper
- 1 red onion

Protein Component:

- 1 cup dry lentils (green, brown, or black)

Fat Component:

- 1 Tbsp. oil for roasting veggies and sweet potatoes (1 fat serving)

Grain Component:

- 2-3 large sweet potatoes

Other Ingredients:

- 2 Tbsp. olive oil (2 fat servings)
- 1 tsp. garlic powder
- 1 Tbsp. red wine vinegar or apple cider vinegar
- 1 Tbsp. fresh lemon juice

- 2 tsp. dijon mustard
- Salt and pepper to taste

Directions:

1. Peel and dice sweet potato and the other vegetables.
2. Preheat the oven to 400 degrees Fahrenheit.
3. Line two baking sheets with parchment paper. On one baking sheet, spread out a single layer of the vegetables, excluding the greens. On the other baking sheet, spread out a single layer of the diced sweet potatoes.
4. Toss all the vegetables on the sheets with a tablespoon of oil and season well with salt and pepper.
5. Put the baking sheet with the vegetables in the oven and roast until they are cooked but still crisp. This should take about 10 minutes.
6. Remove the vegetables from the oven and put in the other sheet with the sweet potatoes. Roast the sweet potatoes until they are soft and beginning to brown. This should take about 30 minutes.
7. Set both baking sheets aside.
8. In a large sauce pan, combine the lentils with three cups of water. Bring to a boil, then reduce the heat and simmer until the lentils are cooked and the water is absorbed.
9. Meanwhile, in a medium mixing bowl, combine the "other ingredients" and mix thoroughly to make a dressing.
10. When everything is complete, measure out 6 ounces of lentils per serving and the appropriate amount of vegetables and sweet potatoes.
11. Toss everything together with a small amount of the dressing.

Southwestern Eggs and Polenta

Number of Servings: Makes 1 Serving

Time Required: About 30 minutes

Components of Each Serving:

- Protein Servings: 1
- Grain Servings: 1
- Vegetable Servings: 1

Ingredients:

Vegetable Component: (These ingredients will be made into a salsa, 6 oz. of which constitutes a vegetable serving.)

- ½ cup white or yellow onion, diced
- 1 clove garlic, minced
- 1-2 Tbsp. of roasted red chili peppers from a jar
- 1 can (14.5 oz.) fire-roasted tomatoes, diced
- ½ tsp. chipotle chili powder
- 1 tsp. ground cumin

Protein Component:

- 2 eggs

Grain Component:

- 4 oz. polenta (sliced or cooked as a porridge using the directions on the package)

Other Ingredients:

- Fresh cilantro, chopped

Additions for Those on Maintenance Plans:

- *Grain Component:* Increase the amount of polenta.

- *Protein Component:* Add black beans to the mix.
- *Fat Component*: Include chopped fresh avocado.

Directions:

1. In a small sauce pan, sauté the onions, garlic, and roasted chilis with just a dash of oil. Saute just until the mixture is fragrant and the onions are translucent, about 5 minutes.
2. Add the rest of the salsa ingredients and simmer on low for 5-10 minutes.
3. Preheat oven to 350 degrees Fahrenheit.
4. Slice the polenta into 14-inch-thick slices and weigh into appropriate serving sizes. Line a baking sheet with parchment paper and place the polenta slices on the sheet. Brush with a small amount of oil and season well with salt and pepper. Bake for about 10 minutes, until the polenta begins to brown. Remove from oven.
5. Heat a dash of oil over medium heat in a skillet. When the oil is hot, crack the eggs into the pan and turn the heat down to low. Cook for 3 to 6 minutes, just until the yolk begins to set.
6. Transfer the polenta slices to a plate. Top the polenta with eggs, and then top the whole thing with the salsa. Garnish with cilantro if desired.

Lentils and Mushrooms

Number of Servings: Makes 4 Servings

Time Required: About 75 minutes

Components of Each Serving:

- Protein Servings: 1
- Fat Servings: 1
- Vegetable Servings: 1

Ingredients:

Vegetable Component:

- ½ onion, peeled, chopped
- 1 carrot or celery stalk, chopped
- 10 oz. raw crimini mushrooms
- 1 jar (24 oz.) sugar-free tomato sauce
- Spaghetti squash, roasted or steamed

Protein Component:

- 11 oz. dry lentils (green, brown, or black)

Fat Component:

- 2 Tbsp. olive oil

Other Ingredients:

- 2 garlic cloves, halved
- 1 ½ cups vegetable stock
- Salt and pepper to taste

Additions for Those on Maintenance Plans:

- *Grain Component:* Serve over quinoa.

- *Protein Component:* Top with toasted pine nuts.
- *Fat Component:* Increase the amount of oil used.

Directions:

1. Dice the onion, carrot, celery, mushrooms, and garlic.
2. Heat the oil in a large saucepan or skillet over medium-high heat.
3. Add the vegetables to the skillet and sauté, uncovered, for about 10 minutes. The vegetables should be beginning to brown at this point.
4. Add the lentils, stock, and tomato sauce to the vegetables in the skillet. Reduce heat to low and cover.
5. Cook, stirring occasionally, for 45 minutes or until lentils are tender. If all the water is absorbed before the lentils have finished cooking, add water as necessary.
6. Meanwhile, roast the spaghetti squash in a 400-degree oven or cook in a steamer. When the squash is cooked, shred it with a fork.
7. Toss everything together and divide into 4 equal servings. Season well with salt and pepper.

Not Really Spaghetti with Red Sauce

Number of Servings: Makes 1 Serving

Time Required: About 45 minutes

Components of Each Serving:

- Protein Servings: 1
- Fat Servings: 1
- Vegetable Servings: 1

Ingredients:

Vegetable Component

- Fresh mushrooms, sliced
- Spaghetti squash
- Sugar-free marinara sauce

Protein Component:

- 4 oz. veggie sausage

Fat Component:

- ½ oz. olive oil

Other Ingredients:

- Italian herbs
- Salt and pepper to taste

Additions for Those on Maintenance Plans:

- *Grain Component:* Add 4 oz. quinoa (cooked) or polenta.
- *Protein Component:* Top with toasted pine nuts.
- *Fat Component:* Increase the amount of oil used.

Directions:

1. Preheat the oven to 400 degrees Fahrenheit.
2. Cut the spaghetti squash in half and scoop out the seeds. Brush it lightly with oil and season with salt and pepper. Line a baking sheet with parchment paper and place the squash halves face down on the sheet. Bake for 25-30 minutes, until soft.
3. Heat oil in a skillet over medium-high heat. Saute the vegetables and veggie sausage in the skillet until they're browned.
4. Shred the spaghetti squash with two forks.
5. Combine the vegetables, squash and marinara sauce, weighing the total (minus the weight of the sausage) until you have an appropriate amount for a vegetable serving.
6. Season with Italian herbs, salt and pepper.

Asian Cashew Zucchini Noodles

Number of Servings: Makes 2 Servings
Time Required: About 20 minutes

Components of Each Serving:

- Protein Servings: 1
- Fat Servings: 1
- Vegetable Servings: 14 oz.

Ingredients:

Vegetable Component:

- 14 oz. zucchini, peeled and cut into thin strips with food processor
- 8 oz. sliced shitaki mushrooms

Protein Component:

- 2 oz. chopped roasted cashews

Other Ingredients:

- 2 oz. peanut butter
- ¼ tsp. hot pepper sauce
- 1 Tbsp. soy sauce
- Juice of 1 lime
- 2 cloves garlic, minced
- 1-inch piece of fresh ginger, peeled and grated
- 2 Tbsp. sesame oil
- Fresh cilantro, chopped

Additions for Those on Maintenance Plans:

- *Grain Component:* Serve over 4 ounces of white rice.

- *Protein Component:* Increase amount of roasted cashews.
- *Fat Component:* Increase amounts of peanut butter, oil or cashews.

Directions:

1. Heat the sesame oil over medium-high heat in a large skillet.
2. Add the mushrooms and sauté for 3-5 minutes, until browned.
3. Add the garlic and ginger and stir until fragrant but not brown, about 30 seconds.
4. Add the rest of the ingredients, excluding the peanut butter, cashews and cilantro, to the pan.
5. Saute, tossing frequently, for about 2-3 minutes until the ingredients are thoroughly heated.
6. Stir thoroughly to combine the ingredients with the moisture released by the zucchini.
7. Stir in the peanut butter and cashews.
8. Remove from heat and separate into two equal servings.
9. Garnish with cilantro.

Savory Chickpeas and Polenta

Number of Servings: Makes 2 Servings
Time Required: About 20 minutes

Components of Each Serving:
- Protein Servings: 1
- Fat Servings: 1
- Grain Servings: 1
- Vegetable Servings: 6 oz.

Ingredients:
Vegetable Component:
- 1 large bell pepper, diced
- ½ red onion, diced
- ¼ cup tomato paste
- Cauliflower (chopped) or peas

Protein Component:
- 12 oz. canned chickpeas, rinsed and drained

Grain Component:

8 oz. polenta, cooked and sliced

Other Ingredients:
- 2 Tbsp. olive oil
- 3 cloves garlic,minced
- 2 tsp. fresh ginger, peeled and grated
- 1 cup vegetable broth
- 1 tsp. berbere seasoning
- ¼ tsp. salt
- ¼ cup fresh cilantro, chopped

Directions:

1. Preheat the oven to 350 degrees.
2. Slice the polenta into ¼-inch-thick slices. Weigh two portions of 4 ounces each.
3. Line a baking sheet with parchment paper and arrange the polenta slices on it.
4. Brush slices lightly with some of the olive oil, and season with salt and pepper.
5. Bake for 7-10 minutes until slightly brown.
6. Heat the rest of the olive oil in a large skillet over medium-high heat.
7. Saute the onion and bell pepper until soft, about 5 minutes.
8. Add the garlic and ginger, saute just until fragrant but not brown, about 1 minute.
9. Add the broth, chickpeas, tomato paste, berbere seasoning, and salt.
10. Reduce the heat and allow to simmer, uncovered for 5 minutes.
11. Add peas or cauliflower, if desired, and heat thoroughly.
12. Ladle the hot mixture on top of the polenta.
13. Garnish with cilantro.

Asian Rice Nuggets

Number of Servings: Makes 2-3 Servings

Time Required: About 40 minutes

Components of Each Serving:

- Grain Servings: 1

Ingredients:

- ½ cup sushi rice
- 2 nori seaweed sheets
- 1 tsp. sesame seeds
- ¼ tsp. sea salt

Directions:

1. Cook the rice using a rice cooker, steamer, or in a pot on the stove using the appliance directions or your usual method.
2. In a dry skillet heated over medium-low heat, toast one sheet of the nori seaweed just until it gets crisp and its color begins to change. This should take about one minute.
3. Add the sesame seeds to the pan and toast for one minute, tossing constantly.
4. Using a spice grinder or coffee grinder, or a mortar and pestle, finely grind the sesame seeds, nori, and salt.
5. Measure 4 ounces of cooked rice.
6. Add a pinch of the seasoning mixture to the rice.
7. Wet your hands slightly and then use them to form the rice into a small ball.
8. Cut the other sheet of nori into strip, and then use one of the strips to wrap around the rice ball.
9. Each ball is a single serving.

Kimchi Eggs

Number of Servings: Makes 1 Serving

Time Required: About 30 minutes

Components of Each Serving:

- Protein Servings: 1
- Grain Servings: 1
- Vegetable Servings: 6 oz.

Ingredients:

Vegetable Component:

- 6 oz. of prepared kimchi from a jar

Protein Component:

- 2 eggs

Grain Component:

- 1 oz. dry quinoa (makes 4 oz. cooked)

Other Ingredients:

- Salt and pepper

Additions for Those on Maintenance Plans:

- *Grain Component:* Increase dry quinoa amount to 1 ½ oz.
- *Protein Component:* Add chickpeas to the grain component.
- *Fat Component:* Add a teaspoon sesame oil to the quinoa.

Directions:

1. Cook quinoa according to package directions and allow to cool.
2. Measure 6 ounces of the kimchi and stir thoroughly into the quinoa.
3. Fill a medium sauce pan with water and bring to a boil on the stove top.

4. Reduce the heat to a simmer.

5. Carefully crack 2 eggs into the water and allow to cook for three and a half minutes.

6. Use a slotted spoon to remove the eggs from the pan, carefully shaking off excess water.

7. Put the eggs on plates and top with the kimichi and quinoa mixture.

8. Season with salt and pepper.

Brown Rice and Squash Skillet

Number of Servings: Makes 4 Servings

Time Required: About 60 minutes

Components of Each Serving:

- Protein Servings: 1
- Fat Servings: 1
- Vegetable Servings: 1
- Grain Servings: 1

Ingredients:

Vegetable Component:

- 1 small yellow onion, chopped
- 1 small butternut squash, peeled and cubed

Protein Component:

- 16 oz. veggie sausage

Grain Component:

- 8 oz. dry short-grain brown rice

Fat Component:

- 2 Tbsp. olive oil, for squash (2 fat servings)
- 2 Tbsp. olive oil, for sautéing (2 fat servings)

Other Ingredients:

- 2 cloves garlic, pressed or minced
- 32 oz. vegetable broth
- 1 tsp. salt
- Freshly ground black pepper
- Red pepper flakes
- 1-2 Tbsp. each sage and thyme

Directions:

1. Cook rice in a sauce pan with vegetable broth, using twice as much broth as rice. Bring to a boil and then cover and reduce heat to low. Cook until all liquid is absorbed and rice is tender, about 30-40 minutes.
2. Meanwhile, preheat the oven to 400 degrees Fahrenheit.
3. Line a baking sheet with parchment paper and spread the cubed squash in a single layer on the sheet. Toss the squash cubes with 2 tablespoons of olive oil. Season with salt and pepper.
4. Place the baking sheet in the oven and roast until squash is soft, about 20 minutes.
5. Meanwhile, in a large skillet, heat the remaining 2 tablespoons of oil over medium-high heat.
6. Add chopped onion and sliced veggie sausage.
7. Saute, stirring occasionally, about 5 minutes.
8. Add the minced garlic and cook until the garlic is fragrant, about 1 minute more.
9. Add 1 cup vegetable broth to the skillet.
10. When the rice is cooked, stir it into the skillet with the onion and sausage.
11. When the squash is finished, stir it into the skillet, too.
12. Add more broth if necessary to reach the desired consistency.
13. Season with salt, pepper, pepper flakes, thyme and sage.
14. Divide into 4 equal servings.

Tofu Hash

Number of Servings: Makes 1 Serving

Time Required: About 45 minutes

Components of Each Serving:

- Protein Servings: 1
- Grain Servings: 1
- Vegetable Servings: 1

Ingredients:

Vegetable Component:

- 1 red onion, diced
- 1 red bell pepper, diced
- Crimini mushrooms, sliced
- Kale, chopped

Protein Component:

- 4 oz. extra-firm tofu

Grain Component:

- 2-3 large yellow or red potatoes

Other Ingredients:

- Cilantro or green onions
- Salt and pepper to taste
- ¼ tsp. sea salt
- ¼ tsp. garlic powder
- ¼ tsp. cumin powder
- 1/8 tsp. chili powder
- 1 Tbsp. water

Additions for Those on Maintenance Plans:

- *Grain Component:* Increase potatoes to 6 oz.
- *Protein Component:* Add black beans.
- *Fat Component:* Add chopped fresh avocado.

Directions:

1. Preheat oven to 400 Fahrenheit.
2. Wash potatoes and cut into cubes or wedges. Line a baking sheet with parchment paper and spread potatoes in a single layer on the sheet.
3. Season potatoes well with salt and pepper.
4. Bake in the oven on the middle rack until the potatoes are just tender, about 25-30 minutes.
5. In a skillet on the stove top, heat a dash of oil over medium-high heat. When the oil is hot, add the vegetables and saute just until browned, about 5-7 minutes.
6. Add the kale and then cover the skillet, allowing the kale to steam for about 2 minutes.
7. Remove the tofu from the package and break it into bite-size pieces with a fork.
8. Combine the "other ingredients," excluding the cilantro or green onions, in a small mixing bowl.
9. Uncover the skillet and add the tofu. Saute for 2 minutes.
10. Pour the seasoning mixture over the ingredients in the skillet. Saute for 2 more minutes.
11. Measure out 4 ounces of the roasted potatoes per serving and top with the vegetable mixture.
12. Garnish with salsa and fresh cilantro or green onions.

Cauliflower and Squash Bake

Servings: Makes 4 Servings

Time Required: About 80 minutes

Components of Each Serving:

- Vegetable Serving: 1
- Protein Serving: 1
- Fat Serving: 1

Ingredients:

Vegetable Component: (Use enough of these vegetables in combination to make one vegetable serving, total.)

- Cauliflower, cored and chopped
- 1 cup corn, fresh or frozen
- 1 jalapeño pepper, seeded and chopped

Protein Component:

- 9 oz. canned chickpeas, rinsed and drained

Fat Component (sauce that contains both fat and protein):

- 10 oz. cooked butternut squash
- ¼ cup raw cashews
- 16 oz. low-fat or skim milk
- ¼ cup coconut cream
- 2 Tbsp. olive oil
- 1 Tbsp. fresh lemon juice
- 2 tsp. sweet curry powder
- 2 tsp. grated fresh ginger
- 2 tsp. garlic powder
- 2 tsp. onion powder

- ¼ tsp. ground nutmeg
- 1/8 tsp. cayenne pepper
- Salt and freshly ground black pepper, to taste

Additions for Those on Maintenance Plans
- *Grain Additions:* Add 16 oz. of diced potatoes.
- *Protein Additions:* Add more cashews.
- *Fat Additions:* Increase cashews or oil.

Directions:
1. Preheat the oven to 400 degrees Fahrenheit.
2. Slice the squash in half lengthwise and scoop out seeds. Brush the cut sides with a dash of oil and season with salt and pepper. Place the squash cut sides down on a baking sheet lined with parchment paper.
3. Roast the squash for about 30 minutes, until it's fork tender. When it is, remove it from the oven and allow it to cool slightly.
4. In the meantime, prepare and weigh the vegetables to make up four vegetable servings.
5. Spread the vegetables in large casserole dish.
6. Scoop the cooked squash from its shell and weigh out enough to make up a vegetable serving.
7. Add the squash to the blender, along with the rest of the sauce ingredients.
8. Blend until the mixture is a smooth puree.
9. Pour the puree over the vegetables in the casserole dish. Put the dish in the oven and bake, uncovered, for 30 minutes.
10. Serve hot.

Really Sweet Sweet Potatoes

Servings: Makes 1 serving

Time Required: About 75 minutes

Components of Each Serving:
- Grain Servings: 1
- Fruit Servings: 1
- Protein Servings: ½

Ingredients:

Grain Component:
- 4 oz. cooked sweet potato

Fruit Component:
- 2 oz. banana

Protein Component:
- ½ oz. chopped walnuts

Other Ingredients:
- Cinnamon

Directions:
1. Preheat oven to 400 degrees Fahrenheit.
2. Wash sweet potato and pat dry. Pierce the skin several times with a fork. Wrap it in aluminum foil and place it on the center rack of the oven.
3. Bake until the sweet potato is completely tender, about an hour.
4. Carefully remove sweet potato from the oven and allow to cool slightly. Remove the foil and cut sweet potato in half.
5. Scoop flesh from the potato into a medium bowl. Add banana and mash the potato and banana together with a fork.
6. Serve topped with walnuts and a dash of cinnamon.

Asian Veggie Stew

Servings: Makes 4 Servings

Time Required: About an hour

Components of Each Serving:

- Vegetable Servings: 1
- Protein Servings: 1
- Fat Servings: 1

Ingredients:

Vegetable Component:

- 1 eggplant
- 1 onion
- 2 bell peppers
- ½ zucchini
- 1 can (14 oz.) diced tomatoes

Protein Component: (Use only one of the following options.)

- 4 oz. extra firm tofu (per serving)
- 4 oz. edamame (per serving)

Fat Component:

- 4 Tbsp. olive oil

Other Ingredients:

- 1 bay leaf
- 1 Tbsp. miso paste

Additions for Those on Maintenance Plans:

- *Grain Additions:* Serve with an Asian Rice Nugget

- *Protein Additions:* Increase the amount of tofu or edamame.
- *Fat Additions:* Serve with chopped fresh avocado.

Directions:

1. Peel and chop the eggplant into bite-size pieces.
2. Dice the peppers, onion and zucchini into similarly sized pieces.
3. Weigh the vegetables and measure out enough to make up four vegetable servings. Include the weight of the tomatoes in the total measurement, but don't combine the vegetables yet.
4. Finely mince ¼ cup of the onion and combine it with the minced garlic.
5. Heat 3 tablespoons of the oil in a large skillet over medium-high heat.
6. Add the eggplant to the skillet and saute, stirring frequently, for about 10 minutes.
7. In a separate pot, heat the rest of the oil over medium-high heat. Add the minced onion and garlic and saute, stirring, just until the garlic is fragrant, about a minute.
8. Add the eggplant, other vegetables, edamame or tofu, and tomatoes to the pot. Add the bay leaf, too.
9. Cover the pot and reduce the heat to medium to bring the stew to a simmer. Simmer for 15-20 minutes, stirring frequently.
10. After 15-20 minutes, remove the bay leaf and stir in the miso paste.
11. Towards the end of cooking, stir in the tablespoon of miso paste.
12. Divide into 4 equal servings and serve.

Not Really Mashed Potatoes

Servings: Makes 4-6 Servings

Time Required: About 15 minutes

Components of Each Serving:
- Vegetable Servings: 1
- Fat Servings: 1

Ingredients:
Vegetable Component:
- 1 head cauliflower, cored broken into florets

Fat Component:
- 1 Tbsp. olive oil (per serving)
- or 1 oz. cream cheese (per serving)

These additions are optional.

Other Ingredients:
- 1 Tbsp. fresh chives, chopped
- Salt & pepper to taste
- 1-2 Tbsp. garlic powder

Directions:
1. Core the cauliflower and chop it into small pieces.
2. Place cauliflower in a large pot and add just enough water to cover it completely.
3. Bring the water to boil, then reduce the heat to medium-low. Cook until the cauliflower is completely tender, about 5-7 minutes.
4. Remove the cauliflower from the heat and carefully drain it well.
5. Transfer the cauliflower to a medium bowl and mash well with a potato masher.
6. Stir in the remaining ingredients, including the oil or cream cheese if desired, until they're well combined. Season with salt and pepper to taste.

Not Really Stuffing

Servings: Makes 4 Servings

Time Required: About 30 minutes

Components of Each Serving:

- Vegetable Servings: 1

Ingredients:

Vegetable Component: (Use enough of these ingredients in combination to make up 4 vegetable servings.)

- 1 onion, chopped
- 2 large carrots, peeled and chopped
- 2 celery stalks, chopped or thinly sliced
- 1 small head cauliflower, chopped
- 1 cup chopped mushrooms

Other Ingredients:

- ½ cup vegetable broth
- Salt and pepper to taste
- ¼ cup chopped fresh parsley
- 2 Tbsp. chopped fresh rosemary
- 1 Tbsp. chopped fresh sage

Additions for Those on Maintenance Plans:

- *Grain Additions:* Serve with a serving of mashed potatoes.
- *Protein Additions:* Add roasted pecans or serve with beans.
- *Fat Additions:* Saute the vegetables with olive oil.

Directions:

1. Heat a skillet over medium heat. Add the carrots, onions and celery and cover. Cook until the vegetables are tender, about 7 minutes.
2. Uncover the skillet and add the cauliflower, salt, pepper, and mushrooms. Sauté for 5 minutes more.
3. Add the herbs and broth.
4. Cover the skillet again and reduce the heat to medium-low. Cook until the vegetables are tender but not yet beginning to break down, about 15 minutes more.
5. Serve hot, as you would serve stuffing.

Stuffed Roasted Peppers

Servings: Makes 1 Serving

Time Required: About 45 minutes

Components of Each Serving:
- Vegetable Servings: 1
- Protein Servings: 1
- Fat Serving: 1

Ingredients:

Vegetable Component:
- 1 large bell pepper

Add a combination of the following vegetables to make a vegetable serving in total weight:
- Mushrooms
- Onions
- Peppers
- Zucchini
- Spinach, kale, or chard

Protein Component:
- 4 oz. sausage, diced

Fat Component:
- 1 Tbsp. olive oil

Other Ingredients:
- Fresh basil
- 2 cloves garlic, minced
- 2 oz. marinara sauce
- Dried Italian herbs (oregano, thyme, etc)
- Salt & pepper to taste

Additions for Those on Maintenance Plans:

- *Grain Additions:* Serve over 4 oz. of cooked quinoa.
- *Protein Additions:* Serve topped with chopped nuts.
- *Fat Additions:* Increase the amount of oil used to cook the vegetables.

Directions:

1. Preheat oven to 400 degrees Fahrenheit.
2. Cut the bell pepper in half, remove the seeds and ribs. Brush the cut side of the pepper very lightly with oil.
3. Place the pepper halves, cut side down, on a baking sheet lined with parchment paper.
4. Roast for 15-20 minutes, just until the pepper's skin is beginning to brown.
5. Carefully flip the pepper halves over so that the cut sides are up, and roast for about 10 minutes more.
6. While the pepper is roasting, prepare and weigh the rest of the vegetables.
7. Heat the remaining oil in a skillet over medium-high heat, and sauté the vegetables and sausage until the vegetables are soft and the sausage is fully cooked.
8. Add the marinara sauce, garlic and greens to the skillet, stirring until the greens are wilted.
9. Remove the baking sheet from the oven and carefully fill the pepper halves with the filling mixture.
10. Return the baking sheet to the oven and roast for 5-10 minutes more.

Squashghetti with Pesto

Servings: Makes 1 Servings

Time Required: About 30 minutes

Components of Each Serving:
- Vegetable Servings: 1
- Protein Servings: 1
- Fat Servings: 1

Ingredients:
Vegetable Component:
- Spaghetti squash, steamed and shredded
- Cherry tomatoes, halved

Protein and Fat Components:
- 1 serving of Bright Pesto

Additions for Those on Maintenance Plans:
- *Grain Additions:* Serve over 4 oz. of cooked quinoa or polenta.
- *Protein Additions:* Serve top with chopped nuts.
- *Fat Additions:* Increase amount of oil.

Directions:
1. Peel the spaghetti squash in half lengthwise and scoop out the seeds. Cut the squash into large chunks, about an inch square, and steam in a steamer until tender. Alternatively, you can bake the squash on a parchment-lined baking sheet at 400 degrees Fahrenheit for 25-30 minutes.
2. While the squash is cooking, prepare the pesto according to the Bright Pesto recipe.
3. When the squash is finished, shred it with a fork.
4. Toss the squash together with a serving of the pesto.
5. Transfer to a serving plate and serve topped with halved cherry tomatoes.

Roasted Root Vegetables (and More)

Servings: Makes 2-3 Servings

Time Required: About an hour

Components of Each Serving:

- Vegetable Servings: 1
- Fat Servings: 1

Ingredients:

Vegetable Component: (Use enough of the following vegetables to make up 2-3 servings in total weight)

- Beets
- Carrots
- Parsnips
- Turnips
- Red onion
- Butternut squash
- Brussels sprouts
- Peppers
- Mushrooms

Fat Component:

- 1 Tbsp. of olive oil (per serving)

Other Ingredients:

- Salt and pepper to taste

Directions:

1. Preheat the oven to 450 degrees Fahrenheit.
2. Peel and cut the vegetables into large, bite-size chunks approximately an inch wide.

103

3. Line a baking sheet with parchment paper and spread the vegetables in a single layer on the sheet. Use a second sheet if necessary.
4. Toss the vegetables with the oil so that the chunks are evenly coated with a thin layer of oil. Season the vegetables with salt and pepper.
5. Roast the vegetables in the center of the oven until they're tender. This should take 45 minutes to an hour.
6. Serve the vegetables hot.

Roasted Tofu

Servings: Makes 3 Servings

Time Required: About 45 minutes

Components of Each Serving:

- Protein Servings: 1
- Fat Servings: 1

Ingredients:

- 1 package extra firm tofu, cubed
- 3 Tbsp. sesame oil

For sauce:

- 3 cloves garlic, minced
- 1 tsp. garlic chili paste
- 3 tsp. fresh ginger, peeled and minced
- 3 Tbsp. soy sauce
- 1 ½ Tbsp. rice vinegar
- 1 ½ Tbsp. balsamic vinegar

Directions:

1. Preheat oven to 400 degrees Fahrenheit.
2. Unwrap the tofu, drain if necessary, and cut into cubes.
3. Place the tofu on a parchment-lined baking sheet.
4. Bake the tofu on the oven's center rack for 15-20 minutes. Remove the baking sheet from the oven and allow the tofu to cool.
5. In a medium mixing bowl, whisk together the sauce ingredients.
6. Toss the baked and cooled tofu with the sauce to thoroughly coat and set aside to marinate for 15 minutes.

7. Heat a large skillet over medium heat, then add the tofu and sauce. Stir fry the mixture for 1-2 minutes.

8. Serve hot.

Roasted Brussels Sprouts and Onions

Servings: Makes 2 Servings

Time Required: About 40 minutes

Components of Each Serving:

- Vegetable Servings: 1
- Protein Servings: 1
- Fat Servings: 1

Ingredients:

Vegetable Component:

- 1 lb brussels sprouts, quartered or halved
- 1 cup shallots or red onions, sliced

Protein Component:

- 4 oz. toasted pecans

Fat Component:

- 2 Tbsp. olive oil

Other Ingredients:

- Salt & pepper
- 2-3 cloves garlic, minced

Additions for Those on Maintenance Plans:

- *Grain Additions:* Serve with mashed potatoes.
- *Protein Additions:* Add crumbled sausage or more pecans.
- *Fat Additions:* Increase the amount of oil used, or add more pecans.

Directions:

1. Preheat the oven to 425 degrees.

2. Cut the brussels sprouts in half. If sprouts are especially large, cut them into quarters so that all the pieces will take the same amount of time to cook.

3. Cut the shallots or onions into long, thin strips or rings, not chunks or small dice.

4. Toss the brussels sprouts, onions or shallots, and garlic together, and then spread the mixture on a baking sheet lined with parchment paper.

5. Toss the mixture with oil, and then spread everything in a single layer on the baking sheet. Season with salt and pepper.

6. Place the sheet on the center rack of the oven and roast just until the brussels sprouts are starting to brown, about 20-25 minutes.

7. Remove the sheet from the oven and transfer the roasted vegetables to a large serving bowl. Toss in the pecans and serve hot.

Roasted Cauliflower

Servings: Makes 2 Servings

Time Required: About 50 minutes

Components of Each Serving:

- Vegetable Servings: 1
- Protein Servings: 1
- Fat Servings: 1
- Grain Servings: 1

Ingredients:

Vegetable Component:

- 1 large head of cauliflower, cored and broken into florets
- 1 red onion, diced

Grain Component:

- 8 oz. cooked rice

Protein Component:

- 4 oz. dry roasted hazelnuts, chopped

Fat Component:

- 2 Tbsp. coconut oil

Other Ingredients:

- 1 clove garlic, minced
- ½ Tbsp. ginger, peeled and minced
- Juice of ½ lemon
- 2 tsp. curry powder
- 1 tsp. garam masala
- ½ tsp. sea salt
- Freshly ground black pepper

Directions:

1. Cook rice according to package directions in a pot on the stove or in a rice cooker. Weigh the rice to make up 2 grain servings and set aside.

2. Preheat the oven to 400 degrees.

3. Toss the cauliflower and onions with half of the oil. Spread them in a single even layer on a baking sheet lined with parchment paper.

4. Season the cauliflower and onions with salt, pepper and garam masala.

5. Sprinkle the veggies with salt, pepper, and a little curry powder, curry powder, and garam masala.

6. Place the baking sheet on the oven's center rack and roast the vegetables until they're tender and beginning to brown, about 30-40 minutes.

7. In the meantime, heat the rest of the oil in a skillet over medium-high heat. Add the ginger and garlic and saute, stirring constantly, just until they're fragrant, about a minute.

8. Stir the seasonings and the rice, then remove from heat and set aside.

9. After the cauliflower and onions are finished roasting, toss them with the rice mixture in a large bowl.

10. Toss in the hazelnuts and serve hot.

Roasted Mushrooms

Servings: Makes 2 Servings

Time Required: About 40 minutes

Components of Each Serving:

- Vegetable Servings: 1
- Fat Servings: ½

Ingredients:

Vegetable Component:

- 1 lb. crimini mushrooms, halved

Fat Component:

- 1 Tbsp. olive oil

Other Ingredients:

- 1 Tbsp. Italian herb mix
- 3-4 cloves garlic, minced
- Salt and pepper to taste

Directions:

1. Preheat oven to 450 degrees.
2. In a medium bowl, toss mushrooms with oil and herbs. Season with salt and pepper.
3. Spread the mushrooms in a single layer in a wide, shallow baking dish.
4. Roast on the center rack of the oven, stirring occasionally, until the mushrooms are well browned, about 30 minutes.
5. Serve hot.

Asian Beef with Broccoli

Servings: Makes 4 Servings

Time Required: About 15 minutes

Components of Each Serving:
- Vegetable Servings: 1
- Protein Servings: 1
- Fat Servings: 1

Ingredients:

Vegetable Component: (Combine these vegetables in a total weight to make up four vegetable servings.)
- ½ white onion
- 1 head broccoli
- 1 head cauliflower

Protein Component:
- 1 lb. beef, thinly sliced

Fat Component:
- 1 Tbsp. sesame oil

Other Ingredients:
- ¼ cup soy sauce
- 1 clove garlic, minced
- 1 tsp. ground ginger
- 2 Tbsp. rice vinegar

Directions:
1. Core and chop cauliflower into florets. Steam it in a pot with ½ cup water for about 5 minutes. Drain and set aside.

2. Heat a dash of oil in a skillet over medium-high heat. Add the garlic and ½ teaspoon ginger and saute, stirring constantly, just until they're fragrant, about 1 minute.

3. Add beef and saute, stirring, until the meat begins to brown, about 3 minutes.

4. Add broccoli and onions and continue to saute, stirring, for about 5 minutes more

5. In a small bowl, whisk together sesame oil, soy sauce, rice vinegar, and the remaining ginger.

6. Add the seasoning mixture to the skillet and toss to coat the meat and vegetables.

7. Saute, stirring, for 5 minutes more.

8. Serve hot.

Shrimp and Veggie Noodles

Servings: Makes 4 Servings

Time Required: About 20 minutes

Components of Each Serving:

- Vegetable Servings: 1
- Protein Servings: 1
- Fat Servings: 1

Ingredients:

Vegetable Component:

- 2 yellow squash
- 2 zucchini squash

Protein Component:

- 8 oz. uncooked shrimp
- 8 oz. mushrooms, sliced

Other Ingredients:

- 2 cloves garlic, minced
- ½ tsp. garlic powder
- 1/8 cup sugar-free marinara sauce

Directions:

1. Fill a large pot with about 8 cups water and bring to a boil.
2. Using a food processor with a spiral-cutting or grating blade, cut the squash into thin, spaghetti-like strips.
3. Drop the squash into the boiling water and cook for 3-5 minutes, taking care not to overcook. The strips should still be slightly crunchy.

4. Heat a dash of oil in a skillet over medium-low heat. Add shrimp, mushrooms and garlic and saute just until the shrimp are opaque and the garlic is fragrant, about 3 minutes.

5. Spray a medium-sized pan with a light layer of olive oil spray and begin sauteing your shrimp, mushrooms, and garlic cloves on medium-low heat.

6. Toss the marinara sauce into the mixture and heat through.

7. Season with garlic powder, salt, and pepper.

8. Serve hot.

Unwrapped Burritos

Servings: Makes 2 Servings

Time Required: About 30 minutes

Components of Each Serving:

- Vegetable Servings: 1
- Protein Servings: 1
- Fat Servings: 1
- Grain Servings: 1

Ingredients:

Vegetable Component:

- ½ head of cauliflower
- 2 bell peppers, seeded and chopped
- Lettuce
- Tomato

Protein Component:

- 4 oz. canned black beans
- 4 oz. lean beef, sliced thinly

Fat Component:

- 4 oz. sour cream
- 4 oz. chopped fresh avocado

Grain Component:

- 4 oz. cooked rice or quinoa

Other Ingredients:

- Taco seasoning mix

Directions:

1. Chop lettuce, tomatoes, and bell peppers. Weigh the vegetables to make up two vegetable servings.

2. Heat a skillet over medium-high heat.

3. Add beef to the skillet and stir fry until the meat is thoroughly browned, about 3-4 minutes.

4. Add beans and peppers to the skillet, and continue to stir fry until peppers are beginning to soften, about 5 minutes more.

5. Season with salt, pepper and taco seasoning mix.

6. Serve over rice or quinoa.

Asian Chicken Wraps

Servings: Makes 4 Servings

Time Required: About 20 minutes

Components of Each Serving:

- Protein Servings: 1
- Vegetable Servings: 1

Ingredients:

Protein Component:

- 1 lb. ground chicken

Vegetable Component:

- 8 oz. canned water chestnuts, drained and diced
- 2 green onions
- 1 yellow onion
- 1 head butter lettuce

Other Ingredients:

- 2 cloves garlic, minced
- 2 Tbsp. soy sauce
- 1 Tbsp. rice wine vinegar
- 1 Tbsp. fresh ginger, peeled and minced
- 1 (8 oz can) water chestnuts, drained and diced

Directions:

1. Separate the butter lettuce leaves
2. Chop water chestnuts, onion, and green onions into a medium dice
3. Heat a dash of oil in a large skillet over medium-high heat

4. Add the ground chicken to the skillet and cook, stirring to break up clumps of the meat, until it is well browned.

5. Add soy sauce, rice wine vinegar, onion, and garlic to the skillet and continue to saute, stirring, until the chicken is thoroughly cooked, about 5 minutes more.

6. Add the green onions and water chestnuts, and season to taste with salt and pepper.

7. Spoon the mixture into butter lettuce leaves and wrap it all up.

8. Serve hot with extra soy sauce.

Desserts

At first glance, the Bright Line Eating plan looks like it spells the end for desserts. First of all, the plan outlaws sugar, and you certainly can't have a sweet dessert without sugar, can you? Then the plan also prohibits flour, and that means it rules out all kinds of baked goods. No cakes, cookies, candies, pastries or any other similar treats. That means no dessert, right?

No, that's not what it means. It means that you have to change your idea about what makes a treat. There are ways to concoct sweet treats without using sugar, and there are ways to create delectable baked goods without using flour.

We've included some recipes here that do just that. We've found meal-ending dishes that hit all the right dessert notes without violating any of the Bright Line boundaries. All you have to do is make sure that you have room for them within your serving-size limits, and then you can enjoy them entirely free of guilt.

Not Really Pumpkin Pie

Servings: Makes 1 Serving

Time Required: About 10 minutes

Components of Each Serving:

- Vegetable Servings: 1
- Protein Servings: 1
- Grain Servings: 1

Ingredients:

Vegetable Component:

- 4 oz. canned pumpkin puree

Grain Component:

- 1 oz. old-fashioned oats

Protein Component:

- 4 oz. low-fat or skim milk

Other Ingredients:

- ¼ tsp. pumpkin pie spice

Directions:

1. In a medium sauce pan, combine oats, pumpkin puree, milk, and pumpkin pie spice.
2. Cook gently over medium-low heat until the oats are tender and begin to thicken, about 5-7 minutes.
3. Transfer to a serving bowl and serve hot.

Peach Cobbler

Servings: Makes 1 Serving

Time Required: About 30 minutes

Components of Each Serving:

- Fruit Servings: 1
- Grain Servings: 1
- Protein Servings: 1

Ingredients:

Fruit Component:

- 1-2 ripe peaches

Grain Component:

- 1 oz. dry oatmeal

Protein Component:

- 1 ½ oz. peanut butter

Other Ingredients:

- ¼ tsp. cinnamon
- ¼ tsp. salt
- Olive oil spray

Directions:

1. Preheat oven to 350°
2. Slice peaches and measure out enough for a single fruit serving.
3. Spray a small baking dish with a small amount of olive oil cooking spray.
4. Place the peaches in a single layer on the bottom of the baking dish.
5. In a small mixing bowl, combine oatmeal, peanut butter, salt and cinnamon

6. Spread this mixture over the top of the peaches

7. Place dish on the oven's center rack and bake for about 25 minutes, until the topping is golden brown.

8. Serve warm.

Dessert Latkes

Servings: Makes 1 Serving

Time Required: About 20 minutes

Components of Each Serving:

- Grain Servings: 1
- Protein Servings: 1
- Fruit Servings: 1

Ingredients:

Grain Component:

- 4 oz. cooked sweet potato

Protein Component:

- 4 oz. low-fat or skim milk
- ½ oz. flaxseed meal
- 2 oz. low-fat yogurt

Fruit Component:

- 6 oz. blueberries or strawberries

Additions for Those on Maintenance Plans:

- *Grain Additions:* Increase grain to 6 oz. sweet potato.
- *Protein Additions:* Top with more yogurt or chopped nuts.

Directions:

1. Microwave a small sweet potato until soft and easily mashable with a fork. This should take 8-10 minutes.
2. Carefully remove the sweet potato's skin, and mash the potato's flesh with a fork in a medium mixing bowl.
3. Add the flaxseed meal and milk.

4. Mix well to form a thick batter.

5. Heat a dash of oil on a skillet or griddle over medium-high heat

6. Shape the batter into a large, flat patty and place on the griddle or skillet.

7. Cook thoroughly on one side, about 2-3 minutes, then flip and cook the other side.

8. Transfer to a serving plate and serve warm, topped with yogurt and fruit.

Sweet Potato Dessert Bake

Number of Servings: Makes 6 Servings

Time Required: About 45 minutes

Components of Each Serving:

- Protein Servings: 1
- Grain Servings: 1
- Fruit Servings: 1/2

Ingredients:

Fruit Component

- 1 ripe large banana
- 12 oz. honey crisp apple (about 2 apples), diced

Protein Component:

- 16 oz. soy milk or low-fat or skim milk
- 4 oz. chopped pecans, walnuts, or hazelnuts
- 2 oz. yogurt for topping on each serving.

Grain Component:

- 2 oz. rolled oats
- 8 oz. cooked sweet potato, peeled and mashed (about 1 large potato)
- 2 oz. rolled oats (for topping)

Other Ingredients:

- 1-2 tsp. vanilla extract
- 1 tsp. ground cinnamon
- 1/8 tsp. nutmeg
- ¼ tsp. salt

Additions for Those on Maintenance Plans:

- *Grain Component:* Decrease the total number of servings to 4 (so that you eat ¼ of the total).
- *Protein Component:* Increase total amount of nuts to 8 oz.
- *Fat Component:* Increase apple total weight to 18 oz.

Directions:

1. Preheat the oven to 350 degrees Fahrenheit.
2. Fill a medium pot 2/3 full of water and bring to a boil. Add whole sweet potato to the pot. Cover and cook until tender, about 10 minutes.
3. Drain the sweet potato and set aside.
4. Rinse the pot and add 2 ounces oats and 16 ounces milk. Whisk together and bring to a boil.
5. Reduce heat to low and cook for about 5 minutes more, stirring frequently.
6. Using a fork, peel the skin from the sweet potato and weigh out 8 ounces. Using a potato masher or fork, mash in the cooked sweet potato in the pot. Add the peeled banana and mash it into the sweet potato. Stir in cinnamon, nutmeg, vanilla, and salt.
7. Put the pot over low heat and cook for 5 more minutes.
8. In a medium mixing bowl, toss the nuts, 2 ounces oats and a bit more cinnamon and nutmeg.
9. Peel and dice the apples.
10. Spread the sweet potato/banana mixture in a casserole dish.
11. Spread the apples in a layer on top of the sweet potatoes.
12. Sprinkle the nut mixture over the top.
13. Place casserole dish in the oven and bake, uncovered, for 30 minutes.
14. Remove and allow to cool slightly. Divide into 6 equal servings.

Conclusion

If you've made the decision to follow the Bright Line Eating plan, it means you're serious about controlling your unhealthy eating habits and losing weight. You've chosen a plan that takes a no-nonsense approach to disciplined eating and that has no patience for deviations or excuses.

Staying with a plan like that is a challenge, but if you can do it, it has the potential to deliver benefits to your life that reach far beyond weight loss. It won't be easy, but the potential rewards are great.

To try to make this challenge as easy for you as possible--and even to help you decide if the Bright Line Eating plan is right for you in the first place--we've gathered all the information and tools that we could find into this book. We've given you the background, the details, the method, the recipes, and the tools to make Bright Line a sustainable part of your life.

The rest is up to you.

CPSIA information can be obtained
at www.ICGtesting.com
Printed in the USA
LVHW100826021219
639121LV00012B/559/P

9 781949 143393